STRENGTHEN
YOUR
BACK

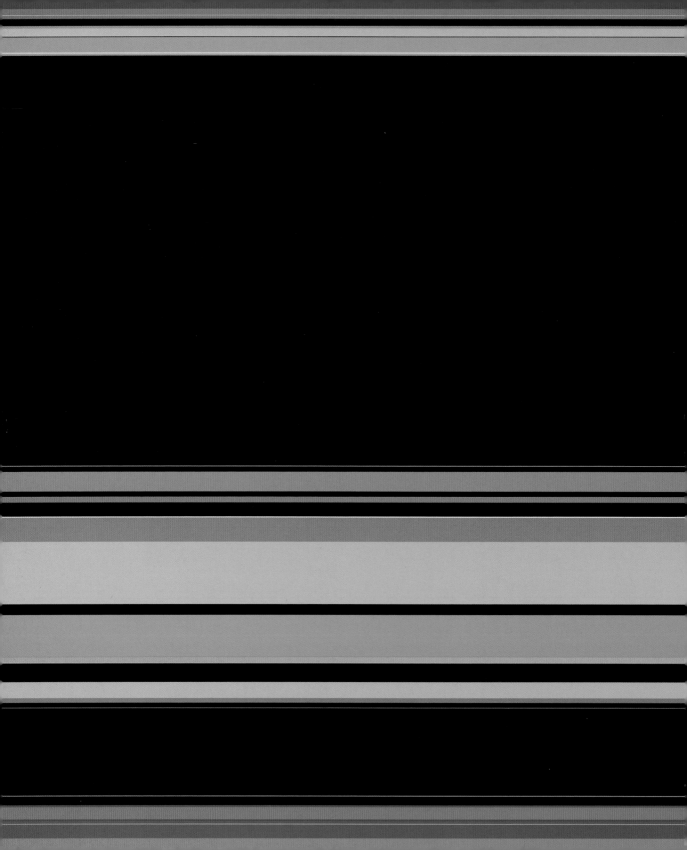

STRENGTHEN YOUR BACK

LONDON, NEW YORK, MUNICH,
MELBOURNE, DELHI

Senior Editors	Gareth Jones, Ed Wilson
Senior Art Editors	Gillian Andrews, Keith Davis
Project Editors	Corinne Masciocchi, Hannah Bowen, Cécile Landau, Scarlett O'Hara
US Editor	Jill Hamilton
US Medical Consultant	Eric N. Dubrow, MD
Project Art Editors	Phil Gamble, Yen Mai Tsang
Production Editor	Joanna Byrne
Production Controller	Sophie Argyris
Jacket Designer	Mark Cavanagh
Managing Editor	Stephanie Farrow
Managing Art Editor	Lee Griffiths
Illustrators	Philip Wilson, Debbie Maizels, Mark Walker, Debajyoti Dutta, Phil Gamble, Darren Awuah

First American Edition, 2013
Published in the United States by
DK Publishing
345 Hudson Street
New York, New York 10014

10 9 8 7 6 5 4 3 2

006–195567–Oct/2013

Published in Great Britain by
Dorling Kindersley Limited.

A catalog record for this book is available
from the Library of Congress.
ISBN 978-1-4654-1455-7

DK books are available at special discounts when
purchased in bulk for sales promotions,
premiums, fund-raising, or educational use. For
details, contact: DK Publishing Special Markets,
345 Hudson Street, New York, New York 10014 or
SpecialSales@dk.com.

Color reproduction by Alta Image, UK
Printed in China by Hung Hing

Discover more at
www.dk.com

CONTENTS

BACK & NECK ANATOMY

DIAGNOSIS & TREATMENT

PREVENTING & COPING WITH PAIN

MAINTENANCE & REHABILITATION EXERCISES

BMA MEDICAL EDITOR

Dr. Michael Peters is Consulting Medical Editor to the British Medical Association and Director of the Doctors for Doctors Unit at the BMA, having previously worked as a GP.

CONSULTANT EDITORS

Dr. John Tanner is a private practitioner in musculoskeletal and sports medicine with a special interest in back injuries and their treatment. He qualified in medicine and psychology in London and trained as a general practitioner, then went on to study medical and osteopathic methods of manipulation, physical fitness training, sports injuries, and pain management. He now runs a multidisciplinary clinic in West Sussex that specializes in musculoskeletal problems (www.ovingclinic.co.uk), is Education Chairman of the British Institute of Musculoskeletal Medicine, and organizes the teaching program for doctors in this field. He lectures for the International Spine Intervention Society in Europe and is Co Clinical Lead at Bupa Health and Wellbeing, Barbican, London.

Eva Niezgoda-Hadjidemetri Msc MCSP HPC is a musculoskeletal physical therapist who gained a Masters degree in Physical Rehabilitation in Warsaw, Poland, after which she worked in Warsaw's Rehabilitation Centre. Since moving to the UK in 1986 she has attended numerous postgraduate training courses in manual therapy, gaining an extensive knowledge of Maitland, Cyriax, McKenzie, and neurodynamic methods. A specialist in the rehabilitation of neck and back conditions, with a special interest in sports injuries and hypermobility syndrome, Eva currently works at the 999 Medical & Diagnostic Centre, London.

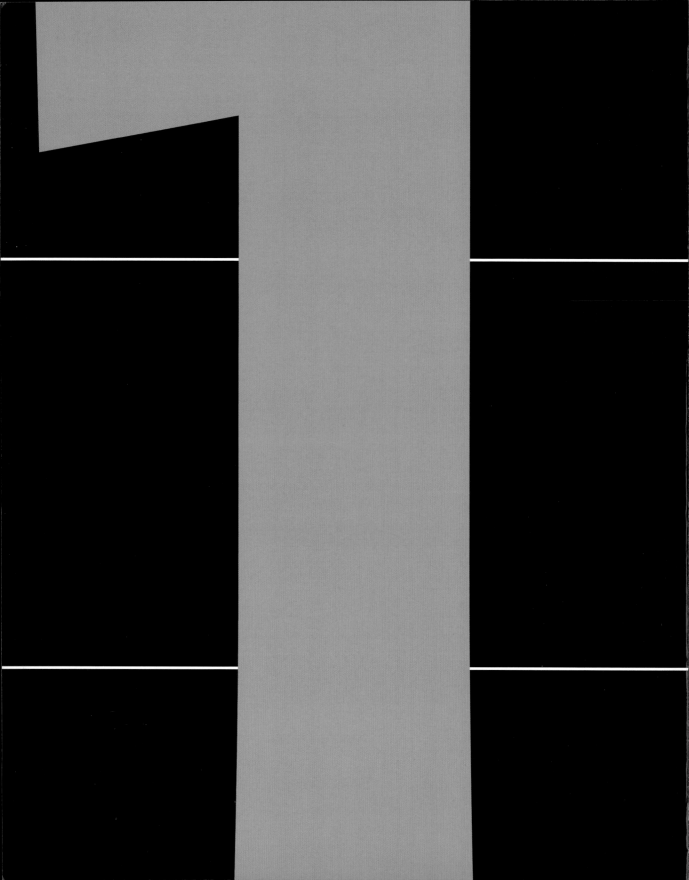

BACK & NECK ANATOMY

This chapter gives an overview of basic anatomy, helping you to understand the structure of your back and neck, and how your body functions. Detailed anatomical diagrams examine the spine and explain how it links up with the nerves, muscles, and ligaments that surround it.

THE SPINE

Your spine is the central support system for your entire body, assisting with nearly all movement, while supporting and protecting your spinal cord. It must be firm enough to support your body weight when standing, yet flexible and strong enough to anchor your body while helping your upper and lower limbs to move smoothly.

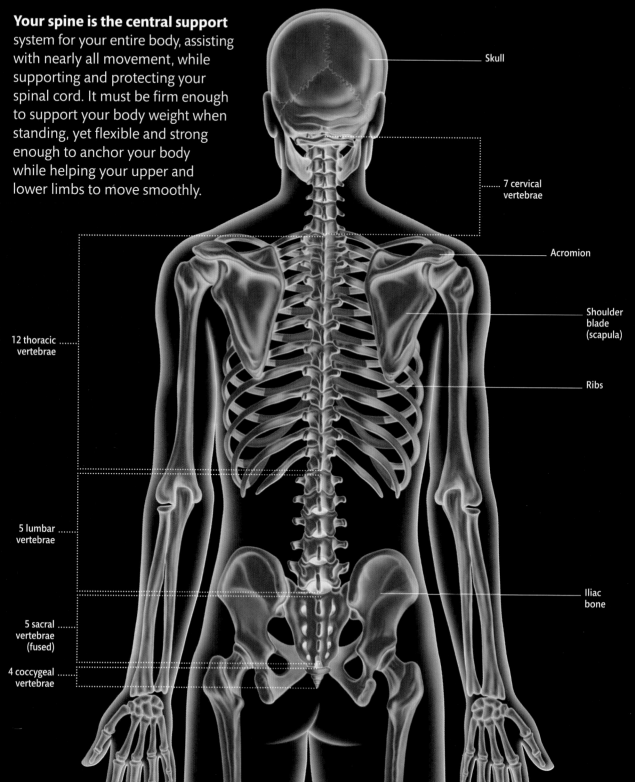

Skull

7 cervical vertebrae

Acromion

Shoulder blade (scapula)

Ribs

12 thoracic vertebrae

5 lumbar vertebrae

Iliac bone

5 sacral vertebrae (fused)

4 coccygeal vertebrae

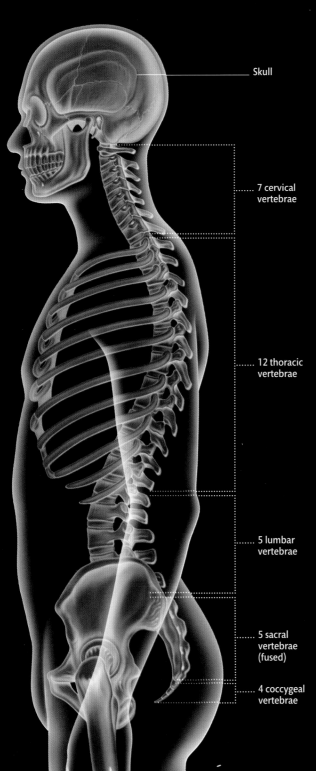

Skull

7 cervical
vertebrae

12 thoracic
vertebrae

5 lumbar
vertebrae

5 sacral
vertebrae
(fused)

4 coccygeal
vertebrae

THE SPINAL COLUMN

Your spine is a column of up to 34 bones called vertebrae. All but 10 of these vertebrae are movable and they are divided into three groups: seven cervical (neck), 12 thoracic (midback), and five lumbar (lower back). The remaining 10 vertebrae are located at the base of the spine; five of these are fused together to form a triangular-shaped bone—the sacrum—which sits between your two iliac bones to form your pelvis. Below this there are three to five (most people have four) fused or partially mobile segments that form your coccyx, the rudimentary "tail" inherited from early human ancestors.

The cervical spine

The seven cervical vertebrae, or neck bones, provide the main support for your skull and allow you to rotate and nod your head. The spine is a mobile structure and can bend and rotate in almost any direction. The cervical region is the most mobile section of the spine.

The thoracic spine

Each of the 12 thoracic vertebrae of the midback is joined to a rib on either side, with the resulting rib cage surrounding and protecting your heart, lungs, and liver. When you inhale fully, the thoracic spine extends slightly as the ribs rise; when you exhale, the thoracic spine flexes. When you twist your upper body, it rotates around your thoracic spine.

The lumbar spine

When you are upright—during most of your waking hours—the five lumbar vertebrae bear the bulk of your weight and provide a flexible link between the upper and lower parts of your body.

The sacral spine

Below the five lumbar vertebrae, the five sacral vertebrae fuse together to form a bone called the sacrum. This bone is noticeably different in men and women, with a man's sacrum being longer and narrower than a woman's. The sacral vertebrae are connected to the vertebrae at the end of the spine—known as the coccygeal vertebrae—by a joint called the sacrococcygeal symphysis. Together, the coccygeal vertebrae form the coccyx, or tail bone.

THE VERTEBRAE

The main part of a vertebra is more or less cylindrical, with a flat surface at the top and bottom, and a small hole running vertically through each, toward the back edge. When your vertebrae are aligned, these form a channel—the spinal or neural canal—that contains and protects your spinal cord.

The back of each vertebra has seven projections, which are called processes. These are arranged in three pairs with an odd one out—the spinous process. Your spinous processes are the knobbly bits that run all the way down your spine.

The spinous process sits between the six paired processes (three on either side). Two of the pairs—the upper articular processes and the lower articular processes—act as joints, linking your vertebrae and strengthening your spine. Your back muscles are attached to the remaining pair, the transverse processes, and also to the spinous process, all of which provide anchorage as your muscles contract and relax.

THE FACET JOINTS

Each of the vertebrae in your spinal column meets at a facet joint. It is here that the lower articular processes of the first vertebra link up, or "articulate," with the upper articular processes of the second. The surfaces of these processes are smooth and flat, like the facets of a diamond—hence the reason that the joints are called facet joints, as well as being known as posterior joints.

STRUCTURE OF THE VERTEBRAE

No two vertebrae are exactly alike. Although they fit together perfectly, they all have individual characteristics. Shown below is a cross section of one of the lowest two thoracic vertebrae, which have small flat facets (costal facets) where they are attached to the ribs, and a cross section of one of the first two lumbar vertebrae, which have much larger processes (spinous processes).

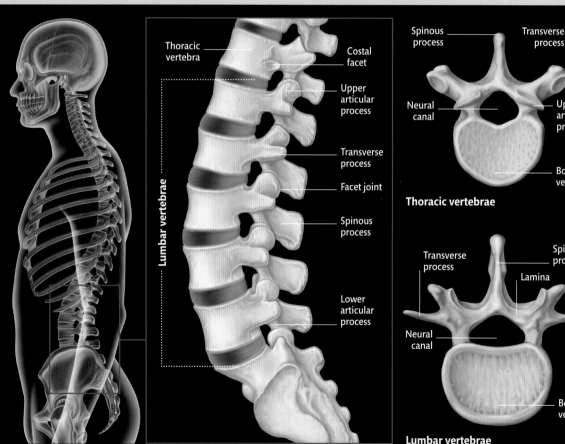

Thoracic vertebra

Lumbar vertebrae

Costal facet

Upper articular process

Transverse process

Facet joint

Spinous process

Lower articular process

Spinous process

Transverse process

Neural canal

Upper articular process

Body of vertebra

Thoracic vertebrae

Transverse process

Spinous process

Lamina

Neural canal

Body of vertebra

Lumbar vertebrae

SPINAL JOINTS

The joints between your vertebrae are each made up of two main elements: the first is a facet joint in which the lower processes of one vertebra balance on the upper processes of the vertebra beneath it to form a fulcrum (**» below**); the second is a flexible disk that works like a moldable ball bearing, allowing your spine to twist and bend, while also acting as a shock absorber.

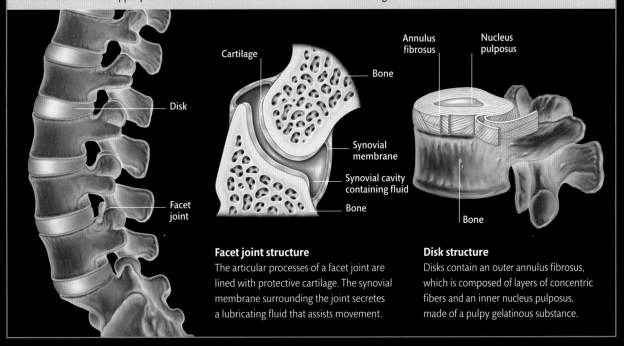

Facet joint structure
The articular processes of a facet joint are lined with protective cartilage. The synovial membrane surrounding the joint secretes a lubricating fluid that assists movement.

Disk structure
Disks contain an outer annulus fibrosus, which is composed of layers of concentric fibers and an inner nucleus pulposus, made of a pulpy gelatinous substance.

The articulating surfaces of the processes are lined with cartilage, while the joint itself is covered by the synovial membrane, which not only forms a protective capsule around the joint, but also produces synovial fluid—a lubricating liquid that fills the cavity and helps reduce friction within the joint. It is important to note that you should perform regular and repetitive movement to maintain the health of this cartilage and keep your facet joints working efficiently.

THE DISKS

The flat surfaces at the top and bottom of the main body of your vertebrae are covered in a thin layer of cartilage known as an end plate. A cartilage pad, called a disk, is positioned between these two end plates, separating each vertebra in your spinal column from the vertebrae above and below it, enabling you to move and twist your body. The outer layers of this disk are made up of bands of tough fibrous cartilage, which form what is known as the annulus fibrosus. The annulus fibrosus then blends with the end plate cartilage, which coats the flat surfaces of each vertebra.

Inside the annulus fibrosus, filling the center of the disk, is a pulpy gelatinous substance. This gel—the nucleus pulposus—allows the disk to mold and reshape itself like a liquid ball bearing. This means that, in addition to acting as a joint, the disk is able to perform a second, equally essential, role as a shock-absorbing cushion between each vertebra.

A healthy disk is extremely strong—much stronger, in fact, than a vertebra. This great strength means that a disk is capable of absorbing considerable forces, or shocks. The disk is also able to absorb compressive and jarring forces with a high degree of efficiency because it can adapt its shape, distributing the strain across its surface more evenly. However, disks are more vulnerable to stresses that are caused by twisting motions—in extreme cases, such movements can cause the outer layers of the disk to rupture. The annulus fibrosus contains a number of pain-sensitive nerves, and the pain associated with a "slipped disk"—a misnomer, since a disk cannot slip, but herniates or ruptures—is often the result of an injured disk pressing on the dural sheath or a nerve, or even from a tear in the fibers of the annulus fibrosus itself.

THE SPINAL CANAL AND NERVES

When your vertebrae are stacked up to form the spinal column, the holes that run through them form a continuous channel called the spinal canal. This both contains and protects the spinal cord, a cluster of nerve fibers that links the brain with all the nerves in the body, carrying signals back and forth.

The spinal cord

The spinal cord runs down from the brain stem, along the spinal canal as far as the first or second lumbar vertebra. A cluster of fine nerve fibers—the cauda equina—hangs down from the base of the cord.

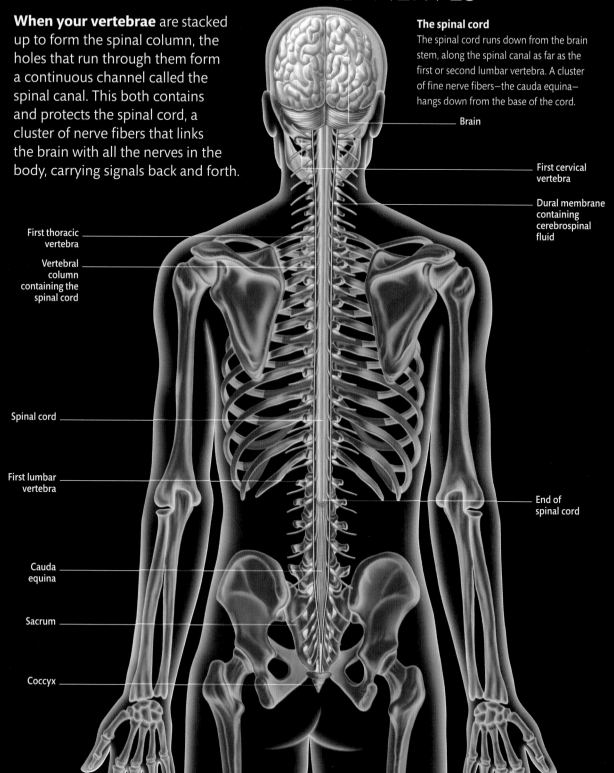

Brain

First cervical vertebra

Dural membrane containing cerebrospinal fluid

First thoracic vertebra

Vertebral column containing the spinal cord

Spinal cord

First lumbar vertebra

End of spinal cord

Cauda equina

Sacrum

Coccyx

THE SPINAL CORD

The spinal cord is a densely packed bundle of nerve fibers, which links the brain with the vast network of nerves that are responsible for controlling all the movements and sensations of your body. It runs from the base of the skull down to either the first or second lumbar vertebra, depending on the individual. Below this point, nerve fibers extend from the base of the cord in strands, forming what is known, owing to its appearance, as the cauda equina, meaning horse's tail.

The three membranes, or meninges, that protect the brain also surround and protect the spinal cord along its entire length. The outermost of these membranes forms a sheath called the dura, which extends as far as the second of the sacrum's five fused bones. At the points where the pairs of nerve roots emerge from the spinal cord through the gaps in the vertebral column—known as foramina—pairs of dural-root sleeves project from the dural sheath to enclose and protect them.

The dural sheath is extremely responsive to pressure throughout its entire length. Both the dural sheath and root sleeves are quite mobile, but bending or stretching movements can cause the nerve-root sleeve to rub against a protruding disk—if this happens, stretching your leg can cause significant pain because the nerve becomes irritated.

Inside the dural sheath, between the two inner meninges, lies the cerebrospinal fluid. This clear fluid bathes the spinal cord and is the same as the fluid that surrounds the brain, protecting it from injury. It acts as an extra shock absorber to protect the sensitive spinal cord from shocks.

HOW NERVES STIMULATE YOUR MUSCLES

The human nervous system is made up of millions of nerve fibers, which transmit electrical impulses to and from the brain. This system allows the brain to control the functioning of the rest of the body. Nerve fibers can be divided into two main types: sensory fibers, which send out signals or messages relating to sensations, such as pain or change of temperature, to the brain; and motor fibers, which relay messages concerned with movement from the brain to the muscles. The movement of the bundles of fibers that make up the muscles—whether they are contracting or expanding—is controlled by impulses from the nerves.

Whenever you decide to bend your arm, for example, the brain sends out a message that is transmitted along the appropriate nerves to your biceps—the muscle in your upper arm. This signal makes the muscle fibers in your biceps contract, which pulls your forearm up, causing your arm to bend at the elbow.

Electrical signals sent from the brain via the nervous system are also responsible for controlling all of the vital bodily functions that keep us alive, such as our heartbeat, breathing, and digestion—all of which involve muscular activity that we are barely aware of: this is called the autonomic nervous system. The autonomic nervous system is comprised of sympathetic fibers—which are involved in fight and flight responses, such as increased heart rate—and parasympathetic fibers, which are involved in functions that occur while the body is at rest, such as salivation.

SPINAL NERVES

These nerves branch off and emerge in pairs from either side of the spinal cord through the foramina, or the gaps in the spinal column between the vertebrae and the facet joints.

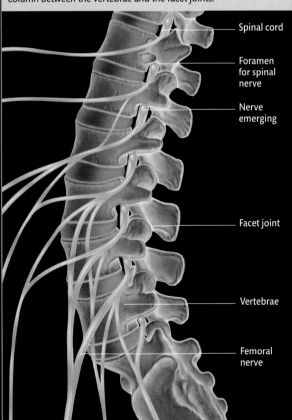

Spinal cord

Foramen for spinal nerve

Nerve emerging

Facet joint

Vertebrae

Femoral nerve

MUSCLES AND LIGAMENTS

The muscles of the back are built up in layers around the skeleton. These muscles are involved with stabilizing and moving the torso.

The muscles of the back
The smaller muscles, shown on the right of the diagram, are mainly concerned with postural adjustment. Layered over these are the larger muscles, shown on the left, which are involved with controlling movement.

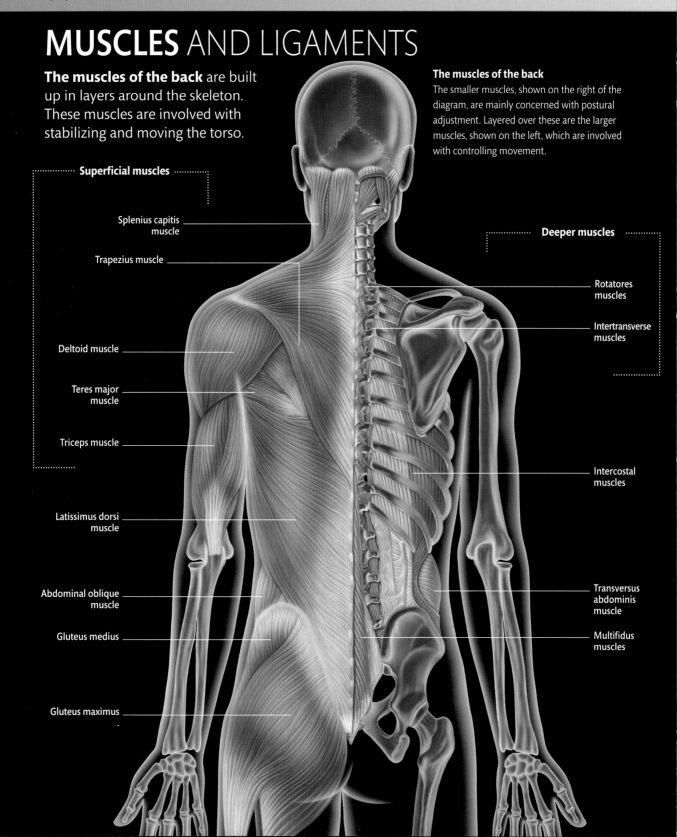

Superficial muscles

Splenius capitis muscle

Trapezius muscle

Deltoid muscle

Teres major muscle

Triceps muscle

Latissimus dorsi muscle

Abdominal oblique muscle

Gluteus medius

Gluteus maximus

Deeper muscles

Rotatores muscles

Intertransverse muscles

Intercostal muscles

Transversus abdominis muscle

Multifidus muscles

THE MUSCLES

Around each spinal joint is a group of muscles. Each end of every muscle is firmly attached to a different bone, either directly or by means of a tough band of fibrous tissue called a tendon. The deeper layers are made up of small muscles that are mainly involved with fine postural adjustment; on top of these are some larger muscles, which are mostly concerned with assisting the movement of the trunk. Muscles usually function in pairs: when a muscle contracts, the opposite muscle relaxes.

The stabilizers

Close to the joints between the vertebrae are clusters of small muscles that contract to allow for subtle alterations of movement. These muscles are known as the stabilizers because of their central role in controlling the positioning of the spine.

SPINAL LIGAMENTS

A network of slightly elastic bands of fiber, or ligaments, helps hold the spinal joints together, keeping the spinal column in one piece and allowing only a limited range of movement in any one direction. Most ligaments contain a large number of nerve endings.

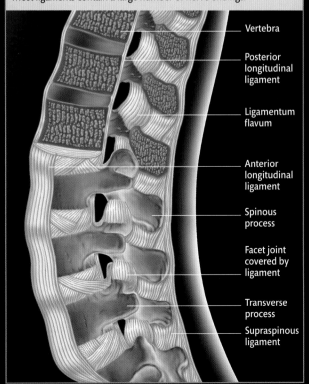

Vertebra

Posterior longitudinal ligament

Ligamentum flavum

Anterior longitudinal ligament

Spinous process

Facet joint covered by ligament

Transverse process

Supraspinous ligament

The mobilizers

These long, strong muscles are superficially visible and control the major movements of the trunk. At the back are the erector spinae ("spine raisers") muscles. They lengthen when you bend over and contract strongly on straightening, exerting significant compressive force on the spine.

Across the front and sides of the body are abdominal muscles that help support your spine by maintaining pressure inside the abdomen and chest. For example, when a weightlifter holds his breath before attempting to lift a heavy weight, he is tensing his abdominal muscles. The transversus abdominis (the deepest layer) works almost continually to assist in performing everyday activities.

How muscles move your trunk

When you twist or rotate your spine, the abdominal and back muscles (collectively known as the muscles of your core) play a key role in the movement. Like most muscles, they work in pairs: when one contracts, its opposite number relaxes. Think of a golfer whose muscles need to create a powerful twisting force to effect a good drive. This force must be balanced by an equal and opposite twisting movement, transmitted along the spine and lower limbs. Over the back muscles lie those of the shoulders and hips. Large, strong muscles support the joints, while smaller, deeper muscles exert a stabilizing force, controlling movement.

Maintaining healthy muscles

Muscles need a good supply of blood. If a muscle goes into spasm in reaction to pain, or becomes contracted due to poor posture, its blood supply will be reduced. If this lack of supply continues, the muscle may become weak and less elastic.

Muscles need exercise in order to stay strong. If they have been contracted for long periods to maintain a certain posture—when you are sitting at a desk, for example—regular stretching will keep them from becoming shorter and weaker. Prolonged pain or even stress can make muscles tense up. Consequently, relaxation is important for maintaining healthy muscles.

Finally, muscles require an intact nerve supply. If an injury or an infection damages a nerve, or its cell unit in the spinal cord, the muscle cannot contract and will waste away.

HOW THE BACK WORKS

The spine supports your entire body—it is responsible for almost every movement you make: you walk not only with your legs, but with your whole back, and you reach for, grasp, lift, and carry objects not just with your arms, but also with your back.

The structure and function of the spine are virtually identical in all mammals. One significant difference between humans and other animals, however, is that during evolution our center of gravity shifted so that, when we are upright, gravity is exerted vertically throughout the length of our body. As a consequence, the human spine, together with its muscles and ligaments, has become a vertical shock absorber, with curvatures to provide the necessary resilience.

The spine must be firm enough to support your body when standing erect, yet strong and flexible enough to provide a source of movement for your upper and lower

limbs. It is structured to allow for a whole host of complex movements, such as bending, reaching, lifting, and twisting. These movements are possible thanks to an elaborate and highly sophisticated relationship between disks, vertebrae, ligaments, and muscles (**≫pp.8–15**).

Between each vertebra is a disk that provides cushioning and absorbs the shock that is created when you walk, run, and move (**≫p.11**). Ligaments—slightly elastic bands of fiber—help hold the vertebrae together, and in doing so allow a range of limited movements in any one direction, according to their length (**≫pp.14–15**).

A group of muscles surrounds each joint of the vertebrae, and the ends of these muscles are firmly attached to a different vertebra, either directly or by a tendon. Close to the joints of the vertebrae, smaller muscles provide subtle alterations of movement when they contract, and it is these that control spinal posture. When you contract your muscles to move your spine, the ligaments and disks, which are specialized ligaments, allow the spinal column to bend.

HOW THE DISK ALLOWS MOVEMENT

If you think of the vertebrae in a spinal joint as two pieces of wood and the nucleus pulposus as a soft rubber ball bearing, as shown, it is easy to see why the disk forms such a mobile joint.

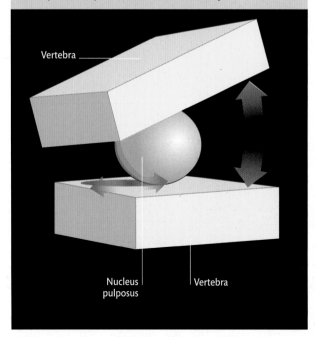

Vertebra

Nucleus pulposus | Vertebra

THE ROLE OF LIGAMENTS

Ligaments extend right down the spinal column to support the vertebrae, hold the spinal joints together, and allow lateral movement.

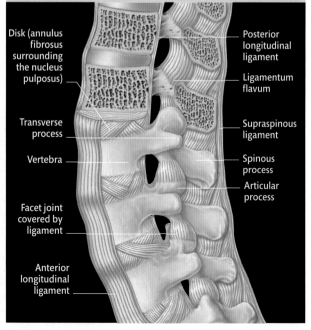

Disk (annulus fibrosus surrounding the nucleus pulposus)

Transverse process

Vertebra

Facet joint covered by ligament

Anterior longitudinal ligament

Posterior longitudinal ligament

Ligamentum flavum

Supraspinous ligament

Spinous process

Articular process

MOVEMENT IN THE BACK

The human spine is the central support system for the entire body and plays a role in almost all our movements. To understand how all the separate parts of the back interrelate to allow movement, it is helpful to divide the spine into three main sections—the neck (cervical), midback (thoracic), and lower back (lumbar)—and look at how each segment functions in relation to the others (»pp.8–9).

■ **The cervical spine** (or neck) is made up of the first seven vertebrae in the spine. It is the most flexible part of the spine because it controls movement in the neck. It must be strong enough to support the head, which is a considerable weight—an adult's head can weigh as much as 14–20lb (6–9kg). It must also be sufficiently flexible to allow you to turn your head so you can look and listen.

At the same time, you must be able to maintain a level gaze so as not to upset your organs of balance: these delicate sensors are located deep in each inner ear and are finely tuned to the forces of gravitation and rotation. This steady gaze is achieved through complex feedback mechanisms in the neck muscles, and these organs of balance allow the brain to account for movement while interpreting visual information at the same time.

■ **The thoracic spine** (or midback), is the longest portion of the spinal column and is made up of the middle 12 vertebrae. The primary function of the thoracic spine is to protect the organs of the chest by providing attachment of the rib cage. However, this function adds bulk that greatly restricts the amount of movement in this portion of the spine. The movements that occur in the midback are limited mostly to rotation and a small amount of flexion and extension.

■ **The lumbar spine** (or lower back) is a more mobile part of the spine. It consists of five vertebrae and lies below the thoracic spine. This section of the spine is a lot more flexible than its neighbor and is the part that you use for many basic activities, such as bending backward and forward, walking, and running. Since it is connected to your pelvis, which is relatively immobile, this is where most of the stresses and strains occur.

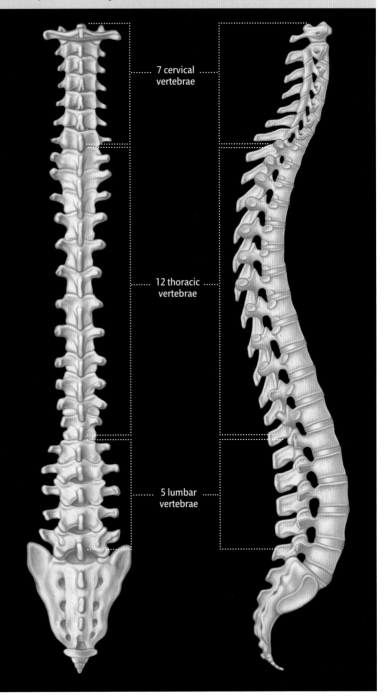

7 cervical vertebrae

12 thoracic vertebrae

5 lumbar vertebrae

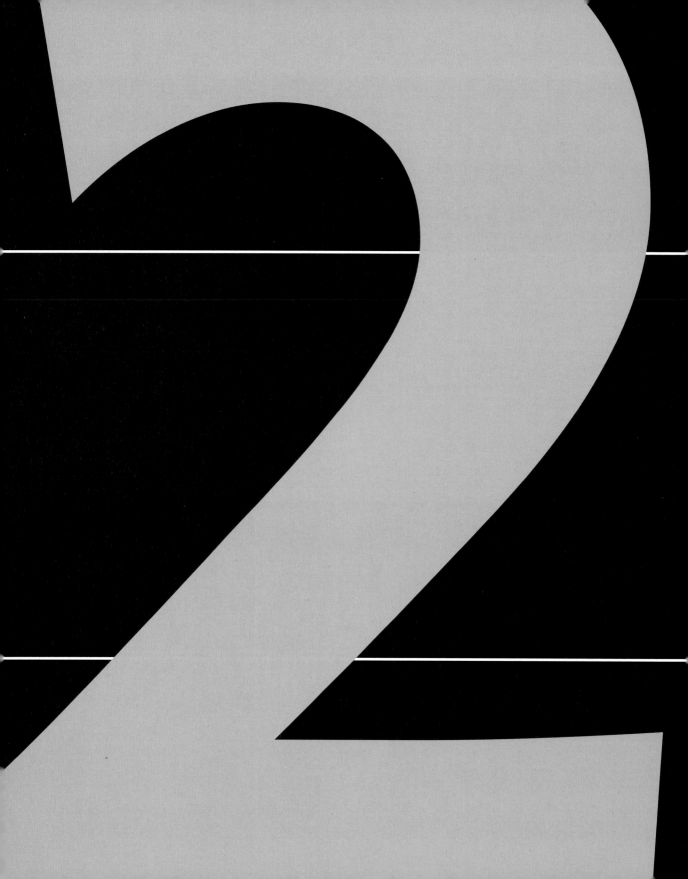

DIAGNOSIS & TREATMENT

Opening with useful symptoms-based diagnostic charts, this chapter offers information on consulting your doctor, a specialist, physical therapist, osteopath, chiropractor, or other practitioner for the treatment and rehabilitation of back and neck pain.

SYMPTOMS CHART: NECK

This symptoms chart will help you determine the potential cause of your neck pain. For further information on unfamiliar terms, refer to the glossary (**》pp.122–123**). These charts are for reference only, however, and you should always consult your doctor for a firm diagnosis.

START HERE

Did your pain develop over the course of a few hours?

NO

YES

Do you have a stiff neck combined with any of the following symptoms: severe headache, rash, nausea or vomiting, aversion to bright light, drowsiness, or confusion?

NO

YES

✚ Seek immediate medical help: could be **meningitis** or a **brain hemorrhage**.

✚ Seek immediate medical help: could be a **spinal cord injury**.

Have you had a violent jolt in the last day or two, such as you might receive if you were in a car accident?

NO

YES

Have your limbs felt weak, or have you had difficulty controlling your leg or arm muscles since this injury?

NO

YES

Is the pain confined to your neck, and did it start no more than a few hours after you sustained this injury?

NO

YES

See your doctor soon: probably a **whiplash injury**, arising from the head being jolted violently back and forth or sideways.

See your doctor: probably **acute torticollis**, literally "twisted neck," which is often the result of sleeping in an awkward position.

Does your neck feel very stiff and painful when you wake up in the morning?

NO

YES

Do you have a severe shooting pain in your shoulder or upper arm that is brought on by trivial movements?

NO

YES

See your doctor: probably a **disk protrusion** compressing spinal nerves, or a **facet joint strain**, which may arise from sudden twisting of a joint.

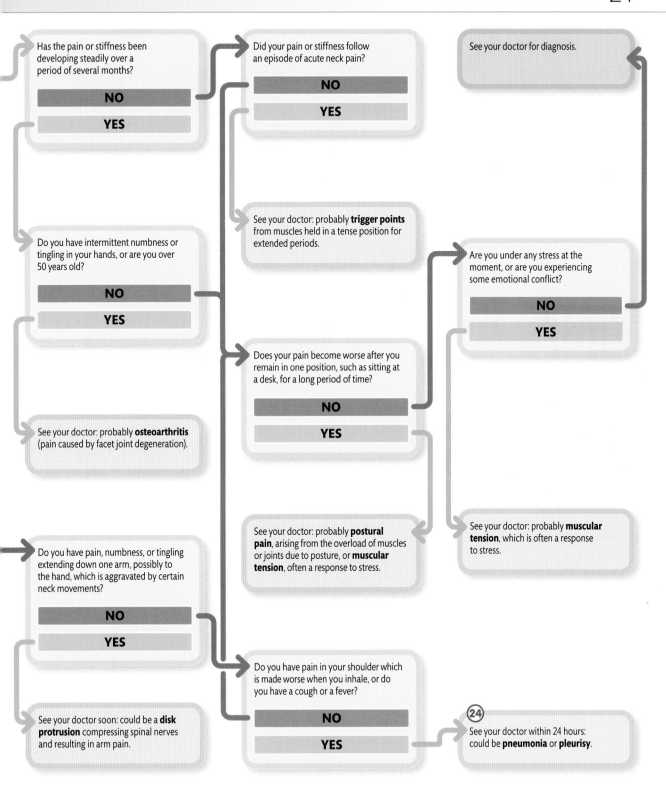

Has the pain or stiffness been developing steadily over a period of several months?

NO

YES

Did your pain or stiffness follow an episode of acute neck pain?

NO

YES

See your doctor for diagnosis.

Do you have intermittent numbness or tingling in your hands, or are you over 50 years old?

NO

YES

See your doctor: probably **trigger points** from muscles held in a tense position for extended periods.

Are you under any stress at the moment, or are you experiencing some emotional conflict?

NO

YES

See your doctor: probably **osteoarthritis** (pain caused by facet joint degeneration).

Does your pain become worse after you remain in one position, such as sitting at a desk, for a long period of time?

NO

YES

See your doctor: probably **postural pain**, arising from the overload of muscles or joints due to posture, or **muscular tension**, often a response to stress.

See your doctor: probably **muscular tension**, which is often a response to stress.

Do you have pain, numbness, or tingling extending down one arm, possibly to the hand, which is aggravated by certain neck movements?

NO

YES

Do you have pain in your shoulder which is made worse when you inhale, or do you have a cough or a fever?

NO

YES

See your doctor soon: could be a **disk protrusion** compressing spinal nerves and resulting in arm pain.

(24) See your doctor within 24 hours: could be **pneumonia** or **pleurisy**.

SYMPTOMS CHART: MIDBACK

This symptoms chart will help you determine the potential cause of pain in your midback. For further information on unfamiliar terms, refer to the glossary (»pp.122–123). The chart is for reference only, however, and you should always consult your doctor for a firm diagnosis.

START HERE

Did your pain build up in just a few hours?

NO

YES

Did your pain start soon after you had received a direct blow to the affected area?

NO

YES

Seek immediate medical help: could be a cracked or **broken rib**, or a more serious **spinal injury**.

Did your pain start after a trivial movement, such as turning over in bed?

NO

YES

See your doctor soon: probably either a **facet joint dysfunction** from sudden twisting of a joint or a **disk protrusion** compressing spinal nerves.

Is your pain sharp, radiating around one or both sides of your chest, and does it get worse when you inhale?

NO

YES

Is your pain severe and constant, and are you elderly or rather frail?

NO

YES

Seek immediate medical help: possibly a **fracture**, which may be caused by age-related weakening of your bones.

Is your pain made worse when you move or change your position?

NO

YES

Do you have a cough, difficulty breathing, any other respiratory problems, or a fever?

NO

YES

24
See your doctor within 24 hours: could be **pleurisy**, **pneumonia**, or **bronchitis**.

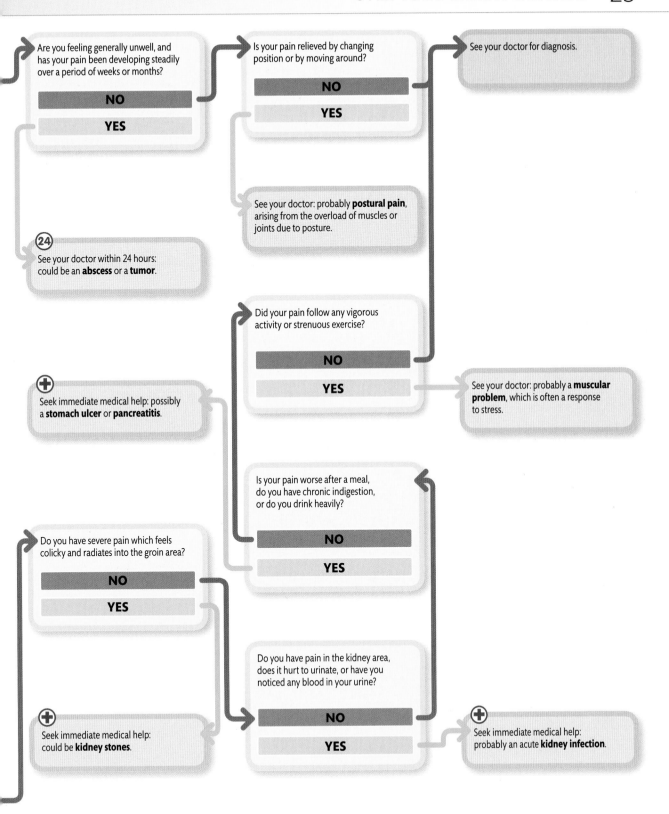

Are you feeling generally unwell, and has your pain been developing steadily over a period of weeks or months?

NO

YES

Is your pain relieved by changing position or by moving around?

NO

YES

See your doctor for diagnosis.

See your doctor: probably **postural pain**, arising from the overload of muscles or joints due to posture.

(24)
See your doctor within 24 hours: could be an **abscess** or a **tumor**.

Did your pain follow any vigorous activity or strenuous exercise?

NO

YES

See your doctor: probably a **muscular problem**, which is often a response to stress.

⊕ Seek immediate medical help: possibly a **stomach ulcer** or **pancreatitis**.

Is your pain worse after a meal, do you have chronic indigestion, or do you drink heavily?

NO

YES

Do you have severe pain which feels colicky and radiates into the groin area?

NO

YES

Do you have pain in the kidney area, does it hurt to urinate, or have you noticed any blood in your urine?

NO

YES

⊕ Seek immediate medical help: could be **kidney stones**.

⊕ Seek immediate medical help: probably an acute **kidney infection**.

SYMPTOMS CHART: LOW BACK AND LEG

This symptoms chart will help you determine the potential cause of pain in your lower back and legs. For further information on unfamiliar terms, refer to the glossary (»pp.122–123). These charts are for reference only, however, and you should always consult your doctor for a firm diagnosis.

Did the pain develop after an awkward twisting or bending movement, or after doing some heavy lifting?

NO

YES

Did the pain develop after a seemingly trivial movement?

NO

YES

See your doctor soon: could be acute low-back pain, probably caused by a **disk protrusion** or **tear**, allowing the disk's soft center to bulge out, or a **facet joint strain**.

≫ **START HERE** ≪

Did the pain in your lower back build up in no more than a few hours?

NO

YES

Did the pain in your leg build up in no more than a few hours?

NO

YES

Do you have a sharp, shooting pain which is combined with numbness or tingling in one of your legs?

NO

YES

Do you have pain extending down one or both of your legs?

NO

YES

Do you have a constant or intermittent pain in your leg, whether or not it is accompanied by any numbness or tingling?

NO

YES

See your doctor soon: could be **sciatica**, caused by a **disk protrusion**, **lateral canal stenosis**, or **piriformis syndrome**.

Is your pain mainly in one buttock, perhaps combined with aching extending down the back of the thigh?

NO

YES

Do you have a pain in your calf muscle brought on by moderate exercise such as brisk walking?

NO

YES

See your doctor: could be **poor blood circulation**.

See your doctor: could be **sacroiliac strain** or **inflammation**, **gluteus medius dysfunction** (buttock muscle strain), or **piriformis syndrome**.

Is your pain mainly in the hip or groin area, perhaps radiating down the front of your leg, and is it made worse when you walk?

NO

YES

Do you have pain or disturbed sensations in both your legs brought on by prolonged standing or walking?

NO

YES

See your doctor soon: could be **central canal stenosis** or **spondylolisthesis**.

Do you have episodes of severe backache with sensations of your back locking in one position?

NO

YES

Is this superimposed on a general background ache, and is it made worse after you have been sitting for a long time?

NO

YES

See your doctor: probably **lumbar instability**, loose ligaments that weaken the lumbar region of the spine.

See your doctor: probably **lumbar instability** or **hypermobility** combined with ligament strain.

Are you middle-aged or elderly, with general backache made worse after activity or during cold weather?

NO

YES

Is your backache combined with any other medical problems, such as colitis, sore eyes, skin rashes, or a urethral discharge?

NO

YES

See your doctor: probably inflammation of the **sacroiliac joints**.

See your doctor: probably **osteoarthritis**, pain caused by facet joint degenration.

Is your backache combined with pain in your abdomen?

NO

YES

(24)

If you are female, see your doctor within 24 hours: could be a **prolapsed womb**, **pelvic infection**, or **period pain**.

Are you under 30, and do you find that your pain and stiffness are relieved by moderate exercise?

NO

YES

If you are male, see your doctor soon: could be a **bowel disorder**.

Are you feeling generally unwell, with little appetite, and are you losing weight?

NO

YES

See your doctor: possibly **ankylosing spondylitis**, a form of spinal arthritis.

See your doctor soon: could be an **infection** or **tumor**, or you may be suffering from depression.

See your doctor: hip joint problem, possibly caused by **osteoarthritis**.

Have you had an operation on your back?

NO

YES

See your doctor soon: surgery may have failed.

Do you have flexible joints, or is your pain worse after you have been standing or sitting for a long time?

NO

YES

See your doctor: probably **postural pain**, caused by strained ligaments or **compressed facet joints**.

See your doctor for diagnosis.

CONSULTING YOUR PRIMARY CARE DOCTOR

If this is your first attack of back pain, you should consult your doctor. Back pain is rarely an emergency, but getting a diagnosis and guidance will help you better manage any future episodes.

Your doctor will probably begin by asking you some, or all, of the following questions:

- Did the pain come on suddenly or build up gradually?
- Where do you feel it, and where does it radiate to?
- Is the pain sharp, dull, heavy, or burning?
- Which positions or movements seem to ease it, and which tend to make it worse?
- Is the pain constant?
- Do you feel any numbness or pins and needles?
- Have you had similar attacks before?
- What kind of job do you do?

DESCRIBING YOUR PAIN

Many adjectives can be used to express the quality and severity of your pain. Some, such as "sharp", "shooting", or "pulsating", may describe the physical sensation; others, such as "gnawing", "burning", or "stinging", may describe your perception of the pain; and others, such as "mild", "moderate", or "severe", may describe its intensity. As different types of pain have different causes, depending on the tissues involved, how you describe your pain will give your doctor a clue to its cause.

A general, dull ache is often the result of tense muscles or irritation deep inside the spinal joints. A sharp, shooting pain is probably due to a pinched nerve and, as with sciatica, you may feel it somewhere other than the injury site.

If you are experiencing a diffuse burning sensation, it is likely to be caused by a problem with your sympathetic nervous system (**»pp.12–13**), which controls involuntary activities such as digestion and circulation of the blood.

DIAGNOSIS AND TREATMENT

After examining you (**»below**), your doctor should be able to make a preliminary diagnosis. Since 94 percent of back pain is purely mechanical, five percent is nerve-root pain, and only one percent has a possibly serious cause that requires further specialist investigation, it is likely that your doctor will be able to offer you reassurance of recovery.

PHYSICAL EXAMINATION

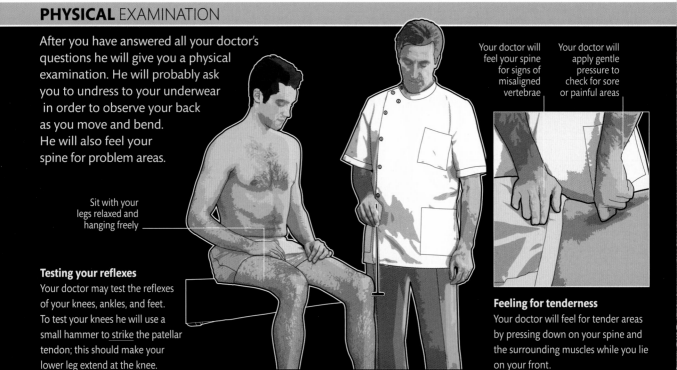

After you have answered all your doctor's questions he will give you a physical examination. He will probably ask you to undress to your underwear in order to observe your back as you move and bend. He will also feel your spine for problem areas.

Sit with your legs relaxed and hanging freely

Your doctor will feel your spine for signs of misaligned vertebrae

Your doctor will apply gentle pressure to check for sore or painful areas

Testing your reflexes
Your doctor may test the reflexes of your knees, ankles, and feet. To test your knees he will use a small hammer to strike the patellar tendon; this should make your lower leg extend at the knee.

Feeling for tenderness
Your doctor will feel for tender areas by pressing down on your spine and the surrounding muscles while you lie on your front.

You may be advised to rest or take it easy for a short period of time while taking simple painkillers or anti-inflammatory drugs, followed by gradually increasing your activity. Your doctor is likely to tell you to be careful not to overdo things, but to stay active and not worry about, or fear, the pain. As you begin to get moving again, you should always bear in mind that "hurt does not usually mean harm." If you have any concerns about how far to push yourself, you can always return to your doctor, or other health professional who might be treating you, for further advice.

If your pain is severe, you will probably need a strong analgesic. Never be afraid to ask for stronger painkillers if you feel that you need them (talk to your doctor if you have any concerns regarding addiction). If you experience recurrent back pain and your job entails lifting or carrying heavy objects, ask your doctor to liaise with your employer about a gradual return to work, with modified or lighter duties.

FURTHER INVESTIGATIONS

If your pain is especially severe or prolonged, or if it recurs frequently, your doctor may suggest further investigations. Initially, you may be referred to a local hospital for a blood test or X-rays, or your doctor's office may have on-site facilities to provide these services. Any further treatment will depend on the results of these tests.

Blood tests

The various tests that are carried out on your blood sample may reveal an infection, inflammation, or even a tumor. They may also show that you are anemic, indicating the possibility of an underlying disease.

X-rays

Soft tissues, such as muscles, ligaments, disks, and cartilage, do not show up on X-rays. Since problems with these tissues are the cause of most back pain, X-rays are often helpful only for ruling out specific causes for your back pain, such as bone damage and disease, tumours, and advanced ankylosing spondylitis.

X-rays can also reveal any degenerative changes that may be present, usually in people over 30, including osteophyte formation and narrowing of the disks or the foramina (the gaps between the vertebrae). However, findings of this type may not always be directly linked to the pain that you are experiencing.

REFERRAL TO A SPECIALIST

If your condition is not improving after 6–8 weeks of treatment from your doctor, you may be referred to an orthopedic specialist. You may be referred earlier if your condition worsens or you develop other symptoms. The first thing a specialist is likely to do, especially if he feels that surgery may be necessary, is arrange for further tests to assess your condition. These may include:

CT scans

CT scanners send out several X-ray beams, each from different angles. This produces a more detailed image than standard X-rays. CT scans show calcification in soft tissues and bone damage more clearly than MRI. However, CT scanning can take up to 40 minutes, during which you have to lie in a narrow tunnel (similar to MRI). It also involves exposure to radiation.

Bone scans

This involves injecting radioactive material into a vein, which is absorbed by your bones, making areas of high tissue renewal—a sign of possible infection, a tumor, or a healing fracture—visible when X-rayed or scanned. The procedure is safe and painless. Problem areas can be detected up to three months earlier than they can via routine X-rays.

Magnetic Resonance Imaging (MRI)

MRI has revolutionized the investigation of problems affecting the spine and musculoskeletal system. It allows the specialist to get a close look at the soft tissues in and around your spine—such as disks, nerves, and the spinal cord—that do not show up on X-rays. During the scan, you are surrounded by a series of large magnets, and the image produced is effectively a photograph of a cross section of your body. By combining these cross sections, a computer can create a detailed picture of your anatomy, clearly revealing muscles, ligaments, organs, and blood vessels.

Discography

This test identifies the exact source of your discogenic pain. You will be given a local anesthetic to let the specialist to insert a long needle into the suspect disk or disks, whereupon a small amount of dye is injected into the center of the disk. This disk is then X-rayed, and you will be asked to describe any symptoms that the procedure provokes. If the X-rays show that the injected dye has spread across the disk and your pain is reproduced simultaneously, it is a positive result if adjacent tested disks are not painful.

Electromyography

By monitoring the electrical activity coming from a particular muscle or set of muscles, both when you are still and when you are moving, electromyography can identify any damage to the nerves controlling those muscles. This procedure involves inserting very fine needles, which are wired up to a monitor, into the muscles that are being investigated in the leg, foot, or calf.

CONSULTING A PHYSICAL THERAPIST

At your first meeting, your physical therapist will carry out a detailed physical examination, look at your medical history, and ask you about your general health and any medication you are currently being prescribed by your doctor.

Your physical therapist will ask you to perform various basic movements, such as walking, standing, and sitting. She may ask you to stand on one leg to assess your balance, and perform more specific movements to help her identify any abnormalities. She may then test your muscle flexibility and strength, and perform neurological and neuromuscular tests, before checking your joints and muscles for pliability and for any problems such as spasms, swelling, or changes in tissue temperature. On the basis of these tests, she will then choose one or more of the following methods to treat your condition.

SPINAL MOBILIZATION AND MANIPULATION

These techniques are used to reduce pain and increase joint mobility, and are often used in conjunction with exercises and guidance on correcting body movements. If using spinal mobilization, your physical therapist will perform a series of movements, with you either in a passive position or actively involved. Spinal manipulation can involve a combination of thrusting movements that are applied to a joint to push it beyond its physiological—but within its anatomical—limit of motion.

THE MCKENZIE METHOD

Your physical therapist will use this comprehensive approach to the spine to identify your underlying disorder. She will guide you through the process, which involves using repeated movements and positions to assess the way your body processes and responds to pain, and help you actively

ASSESSMENT BY A PHYSICAL THERAPIST

Your physical therapist will assess how you use your body and evaluate how your pain is affected by underlying genetic and age-related factors, alongside the effect of everyday movements, and what you can do to avoid aggravating the pain. This involves your physical therapist assessing your muscle length and balance, and how your muscles work together.

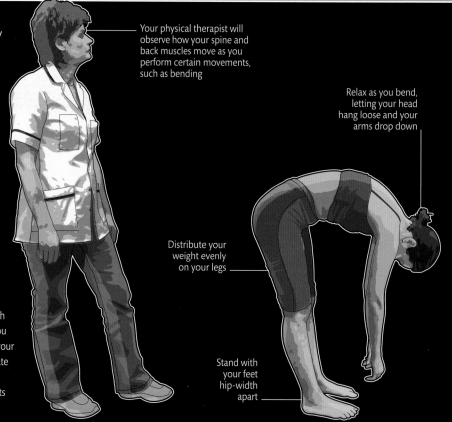

Your physical therapist will observe how your spine and back muscles move as you perform certain movements, such as bending

Relax as you bend, letting your head hang loose and your arms drop down

Distribute your weight evenly on your legs

Stand with your feet hip-width apart

Checking your flexibility
By closely observing your posture—both standing and sitting—and how easily you perform a range of basic movements, your physical therapist will be able to evaluate your condition and flexibility. She may ask you to perform bending movements forward, backward, and to either side.

manage your pain. She will also use the McKenzie method to help you "centralize" the pain in your lower back or neck, even if it initially extends to another part of your body. The aim is to reduce the range of your pain until it disappears altogether, while the new skills and behavior patterns you learn will minimize the risk of recurrence.

SOFT-TISSUE MOBILIZATION

Most physical therapists also employ a wide range of soft-tissue mobilization techniques. Soft tissue refers to all tissue other than bone: tendons, ligaments, fascia, skin, fibrous tissues, synovial membranes, muscle, nerves, and blood vessels.

MYOFASCIAL TRIGGER POINT THERAPY

This involves your physical therapist locating and deactivating painful trigger points (muscle "knots") using manipulation techniques from firm pressure to myofascial release (deep tissue work), often combined with Muscle-Energy Technique and Proprioceptive Neuromuscular Facilitation (»p.30).

THE SCHROTH METHOD

A system of therapeutic exercises designed to correct abnormal curvature of the spine, the Schroth Method was devised by the physical therapist Katharina Schroth (1894–1985) and developed further by her daughter Christa Lehnert-Schroth. It has been used in Germany since 1921, and by the 1960s was the standard nonsurgical treatment for scoliosis in the country. German orthopedic specialists routinely refer scoliosis patients for Schroth treatment. Access to a physical therapist who is trained to offer this type of therapy is often limited in other countries, although its availability is beginning to match the growing demand.

Muscle control

Schroth treatment is based on the idea that the muscles associated with the spine need to be retrained so that they are strong enough to pull it back into its normal vertical position. The exercises are tailored to the individual and are performed in front of a mirror so that patients learn to control their corrected posture. Special breathing exercises enable their ribs to act as levers, assisting their strengthened muscles and helping increase lung capacity.

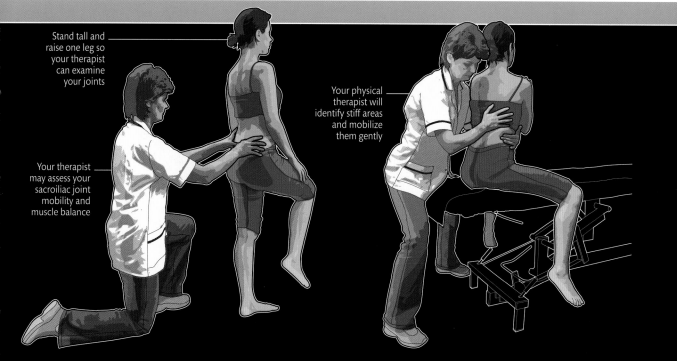

Stand tall and raise one leg so your therapist can examine your joints

Your therapist may assess your sacroiliac joint mobility and muscle balance

Your physical therapist will identify stiff areas and mobilize them gently

Palpation
Your physical therapist will ask you to stand, sit, or lie down, while she palpates (feels) your muscles and joints to assess your movement, muscle action, and pliability. She will also check for signs of poor balance, control of posture, and joint dysfunction.

Assessing segmented mobility
You may be asked to move your body in different directions. Your therapist will feel for any restrictions and check the range of your movements. This can also be used as a mobilizing technique to help you restore the rotational mobility of your spine.

MUSCLE ENERGY TECHNIQUE

This is used to treat somatic dysfunctions, such as impaired movement or muscles in spasm. Your therapist will ask you to perform movements against his resistance, away from the limit of the range of movement, in order to restore full mobility.

PROPRIOCEPTIVE NEUROMUSCULAR FACILITATION

This involves passive and active techniques that your therapist may use to improve the flexibility, coordination, stability, and mobility of your joints, muscles, and other connective tissues.

NEURODYNAMICS OR NEUROMOBILIZATION

This technique is used to treat disorders that involve your nerves, such as sciatica, with the aim of decompressing and mobilizing the affected nerves. It involves a combination of targeted stretching, mobilization, and the correction of your movements.

THERAPEUTIC ULTRASOUND

Your physical therapist may use ultrasound for a range of reasons, such as to increase blood flow, reduce muscle spasm, and speed up the healing of affected cells.

FUNCTIONAL TRAINING

Predominantly using weight-bearing activities, functional training targets the core muscles of your lower back and abdomen. Your therapist will tailor a set of exercises to build up your strength and mobility, and decrease your chances of injury.

SENSORIMOTOR TRAINING

This type of training is primarily concerned with your balance and postural control, and is used in the treatment of chronic musculoskeletal pain. Your physical therapist will guide you through a range of static, dynamic, and functional stages to restore, or improve, nerve-signal communication between your brain and your muscles.

NEUROSTIMULATION

This treatment uses electricity to stimulate the large nerve fibers that block the passage of pain messages to the brain, as well as reducing the action of the small fibers that relay pain messages to the brain from an injury or problem site. It also increases the level of endorphins and encephalins, pain-relieving hormones that circulate around the cerebrospinal fluid in the spinal canal.

TREATMENT

Your physical therapist may employ a wide range of different devices and techniques, in conjunction with hands-on manipulation, to treat the problems you are experiencing with your back and neck.

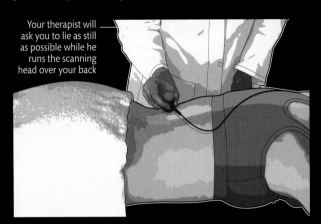

Your therapist will ask you to lie as still as possible while he runs the scanning head over your back

Therapeutic ultrasound
Your therapist will apply a water-based gel to the affected area and will move the therapeutic ultrasound head in a circular motion for about 5 minutes. The ultrasound will encourage the increased generation of new tissues to stimulate repair.

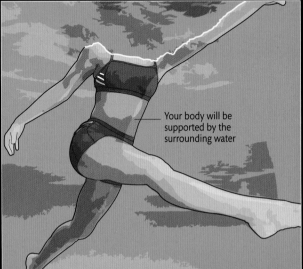

Your body will be supported by the surrounding water

Hydrotherapy
If you have musculoskeletal problems, exercise can improve your condition, but care needs to be taken to avoid damaging yourself further. Performing exercises in water is ideal as your weight is supported, so any stress and strain resulting from your activity will be minimized.

CONSULTING AN OSTEOPATH

Osteopaths adopt a holistic approach to treatment, focusing not only on relieving your back and neck pain, but also on improving your overall health and general level of fitness.

Your osteopath may use a range of different manipulation techniques, some of which may be used together. All of them will be aimed at correcting the problems with your muscles and joints that he considers related to the pain you are feeling. Your osteopath may also give you advice on your diet and exercises aimed at improving your posture.

Osteopathy for treating spinal disorders focuses largely on improving or correcting any abnormal joint movement that a particular injury, or other problem, has caused. Manipulation is aimed at loosening and freeing, rather than realigning, a faulty joint, and it includes rhythmic mobilizing of the joints to restore the optimal range of movement. Your osteopath may also massage an affected area to help relax the muscles there, relieving some of the pain and discomfort before beginning manipulation.

DIAGNOSIS AND TREATMENT

After taking a full medical history, discussing your symptoms, and perhaps performing an assessment of your posture, your osteopath will carry out a thorough physical examination. You will be asked to bend forward, backward, and to either side, describing any pain or discomfort that these movements provoke.

By observing the type of movements that cause you pain, your osteopath will be able to work out which part of your spine is malfunctioning. He may then devise a program of treatment to restore normal pain-free movement. This is likely to involve several sessions of treatment, supported by therapeutic exercises performed at home.

CONSULTING A CHIROPRACTOR

A chiropractor can manipulate your spine to help relieve the back pain caused by different types of spinal disorders.

Chiropractic treatment is based on the theory that mechanical problems with your musculoskeletal system, especially the spine, can affect the way your nerves function, which can lead to a variety of health problems. The nerves that branch out from your spinal cord reach into every part of your body, carrying messages from the brain that control and coordinate all your movements and body functions. If your spinal vertebrae move out of alignment for some reason, the nerve roots next to them can become pinched or trapped, so that they and the parts of your body they control cease to function fully.

Chiropractors use similar methods and techniques to osteopaths and regard back problems as symptoms of problems with the way your entire musculoskeletal system is working. However, they differ from osteopaths in that they focus their treatment on correcting misalignments of the vertebrae that make up your spinal column and relieving any pressure on your nerve roots. The treatment is not painful but there may be some mild discomfort.

DIAGNOSIS AND TREATMENT

Individual chiropractors vary in their approach, but a chiropractic practitioner will always start by taking a full medical history from you, including details of any previous treatment you may have had, followed by checks on your blood pressure, muscle reflexes, and the flexibility of your spine. Your chiropractor may also take X-rays of your back to help detect any misaligned vertebrae or other structural problems.

Your chiropractor may give you remedial exercises to do at home and advise you on posture and back care. You are likely to feel some relief after your first visit, but you may need at least 2–3 sessions before you start to feel the long-term benefits: if you still do not experience any relief, then this treatment is probably not appropriate for your back pain.

OTHER TREATMENTS

A number of other treatments are available to manage and relieve back pain. These range from massage and Alexander Technique to acupuncture, various relaxation techniques, and less orthodox therapies such as aromatherapy and reflexology.

Whatever the actual cause of your back or neck pain, you will almost certainly experience a psychological effect of some kind, especially if your pain is chronic. While there are a number of coping strategies that you can implement yourself, many people find that talking with a therapist can help.

The term "talking therapies" encompasses psychoanalysis, counseling, and Cognitive Behavioral Therapy (CBT). An increasingly popular practice, CBT is a practical, humanistic therapy, in which you and your therapist will uncover, examine, and talk through any negative thought patterns and irrational fears you may have and help you break free from them. The emphasis is on learning to cope, and on developing strategies to help you do this—by accepting your present limitations and working within them—therefore enabling you to regain control of your body and manage your pain effectively.

If you decide to use complementary or alternative medicine, it is important to consult your doctor first, especially if you have a preexisting health condition or are pregnant. You will then need to find a practitioner who will carry out treatment in a way that is suitable for you. Check whether your practitioner is registered with a professional association for their therapy in your own country, although for some therapies there may be no statutory or regulatory body. Any good practitioner should be happy to answer questions about their qualifications and experience.

TREATMENT	WHY CHOOSE IT?	WHAT DOES IT INVOLVE?
Massage	Massage therapy is a very effective treatment for the type of back and neck pain that is triggered by muscular tension. Massages relax the muscles and stimulate circulation of the blood. When a contracted, tense muscle is massaged, the blood flow is increased, and this in turn helps lubricate and soothe the muscle fibers. Tight muscles gradually affect the skeletal system by putting excessive tension on the adjacent bones and joints. Massage helps lengthen the muscles and eliminate any abnormal tension.	You may choose to visit a professional therapist, but even a friend or partner can give you a soothing massage. They should use firm, rhythmic strokes to massage your back or neck, making and breaking contact smoothly and gently while concentrating on the areas of muscle that seem most tense. If you suffer from pain in one particular area, ask the person massaging you to focus on that area. They should work from the top of the spine downward, starting with long strokes from the shoulders down to the middle of the back, or starting from the middle and working down to the buttocks.
Acupuncture	Acupuncture can be an effective treatment for certain conditions such as lower-back pain. It is based on the idea that energy, or "chi," flows through your body in channels called meridians that can become "blocked," making you ill. Practitioners believe that treatment can help restore the flow of chi. You may want to consider acupuncture for the following reasons: to resolve an acute episode of pain; to reduce pain and inflammation arising from osteoarthritis; if you have chronic back pain or sciatica; if chronic "pain patterns" have set in; acupuncture may help break the cycle.	The treatment involves inserting needles into specific points of your body, or trigger points. This may bring relief from long-standing pain and help improve your mobility. Acupuncture works best when combined with physical therapy, as it reduces pain, enabling other methods to balance the body and restore function. There is no guarantee of relief, but patients with a positive attitude toward the treatment are thought to get the best results. Try to find a licensed acupuncturist with a good background of training and experience, who is also medically qualified and registered with a recognized administrative body, and follows recognized hygiene practices.

TREATMENT	WHY CHOOSE IT?	WHAT DOES IT INVOLVE?
Relaxation techniques	Learning to relax completely, regardless of the stresses and strains of your everyday life, could be the key to banishing your back pain forever. There are a number of techniques, including meditation, hypnotherapy, and autogenic training, that will teach you to recognize and reduce muscular tension, and most can be learned fairly quickly and easily. In some cases, the methods can be successfully learned without needing a specialist therapist or teacher to assist you. For example, you may find it easy to master some basic meditation techniques by simply reading about them and trying them out at home. However, you are more likely to get useful results from meditation if you learn a specific method from someone who has been teaching and practising meditation for years. With hypnotherapy, it is best to start by having several sessions with an experienced medical hypnotist.	■ **Meditation** The aim of meditation is to control your mind and focus it to free yourself from stressful fears and emotions. It can also lower your heartbeat and respiration rate. If you have recurrent, mild to moderate back pain that is caused partly by muscular tension, this may help you loosen up, both emotionally and physically. If you have severe back pain, however, it may not be the best choice. ■ **Hypnotherapy** Hypnosis can help influence the way that you perceive your pain. Under hypnosis your control over your conscious mind is suspended so that you are more open to new ideas and ways of processing feelings and sensations as suggested to you by your hypnotist, who can help you enter a state of deep relaxation, in which your pain subsides or vanishes completely. Hypnosis usually works best on people who find it fairly easy to relax, let go of their concerns and worries, and put their trust in others. ■ **Autogenic training** One of the most popular relaxation techniques, autogenic training involves sitting in a relaxed position while you silently repeat designated phrases, using them to stimulate visualizations. This prompts your body and mind to switch off from day-to-day concerns and to focus on calming thoughts, promoting deep relaxation and the release of pent-up tension.
The Alexander Technique	The Alexander Technique aims to treat and prevent a range of disorders by improving posture. It is based on the principle of relaxing muscles—the neck and shoulder muscles in particular—and of adopting the posture that puts the least amount of stress on your spine. A course will not cure acute problems, such as a disk prolapse or acute facet dysfunction, but can help with "trapped nerves" by making more space. However, once an acute attack is over, the technique helps prevent a recurrence. It is especially useful for avoiding postural pain, and if you are elderly, it may prevent acute episodes of back pain by teaching you to use your back properly.	A qualified Alexander teacher will help you undo any postural habits that have become second nature. She will teach you techniques developed specifically for your own posture, which you should practice every day. Your Alexander teacher will help you eliminate postural defects by studying the way you sit, stand, and move. Your teacher will then tailor the lesson accordingly and may work with you sitting, standing, or lying down, depending on what she feels is required. She will encourage you to imagine that you are being pulled upward from the crown of your head. The course may last just a few weeks or up to a year.
Complementary therapies	The therapeutic options for back pain are hugely varied, and include practices designed to tackle not just physical problems, but also psychological ones. Both aromatherapy and reflexology are used to treat back pain, although there is little evidence for their efficacy.	■ **Aromatherapy** Aromatherapy uses essential oils, which are either inhaled or massaged into the skin; the effect is varied, from relaxing and calming to energizing and uplifting. ■ **Reflexology** Reflexologists apply pressure and massage-like techniques to specific points on the hands and feet, known as "reflex points," which they believe correspond to different parts of the body. Easing these is thought to have a beneficial effect on the area in which you are experiencing pain.

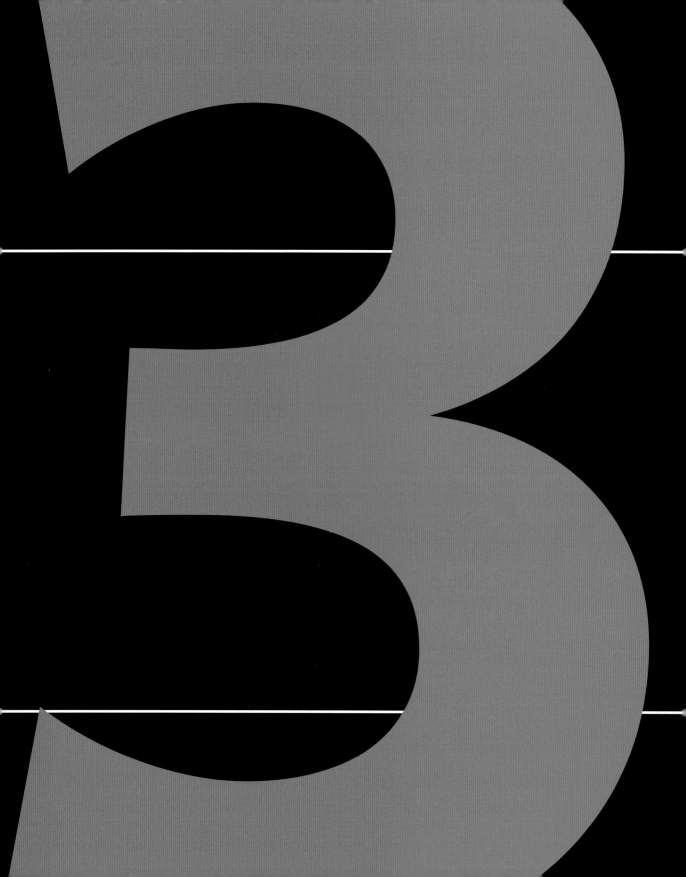

PREVENTING & COPING WITH PAIN

Day in and day out, you may perform any number of movements without a second thought that involve your back and neck. Over time, however, poor posture or incorrectly performed movements can cause or exacerbate back and neck conditions, whether in the form of a sudden twinge or long-term chronic joint damage. This chapter guides you through a range of common activities at work and home, showing you the correct position or movement for each.

IMPROVING YOUR POSTURE

There is no single ideal posture, since humans come in all shapes and sizes. The ideal posture for you is one in which your back is put under the least strain, and in which your spine is naturally and gracefully curved.

Whether you are standing or sitting, the muscles in your back should be relaxed without being slack, and your spine should be gently S-shaped.

GOOD STANDING POSTURE

How you stand and hold yourself makes a big difference not only to the way you look but also to the way you feel. When standing, your body should look symmetrical: it should be aligned equally both side-to-side and back-to-front (**»right**). Correct posture imposes less stress on the spine, so wear and tear is minimized.

The essence of good posture is awareness of fitness. Exercising and stretching your muscles, maintaining good core stability, and how you use your body when still or moving will also help. Fitness helps you stay mentally and emotionally balanced, which will help you avoid tensing your muscles and can help to improve your posture.

BAD STANDING POSTURE

In the context of back pain, posture is poor when it puts your spine under unnecessary strain. Although "poor posture" is generally used to mean slack posture, an excessively rigid posture can be equally bad for your back (**»right**). This results in tense muscles and may even restrict your breathing. Poor posture causes tension in various parts of your body, and your back is more vulnerable to injuries and back pain because your back muscles, ligaments, disks, and spinal joints are all put under extra stress.

CORRECTING BAD POSTURE

If you suffer from aching shoulders and neck, relax these muscles and avoid hunching or tensing. If you are overweight, it increases the stress on your spine because it causes your pelvis to tilt forward unnaturally and moves your center of gravity farther forward. As a result, your back muscles have to work harder, increasing the compression in your lower back. It is therefore important to lose weight and strengthen the muscles of your core.

If you are struggling to stick to a diet, try to do more exercise, perhaps by walking or cycling to work rather than driving. As you start to lose weight, your posture will improve. Do not be tempted to use a corset—it is no substitute for exercise.

If you are pregnant, your growing baby's extra weight will put an additional load on your spine, so good posture is imperative. Keep your abdomen pulled in to reduce the curvature in your lower back and pull in your buttocks so that your center of gravity is over your hips. Avoid locking your knees when standing, which can increase the amount of curvature in your lower back, leading to lower-back pain.

Poor posture can also be caused by foot and ankle irregularities, but these may be corrected with orthotics (**»opposite**). You should also avoid wearing high heels, which can increase the curve of your spine and cause back pain.

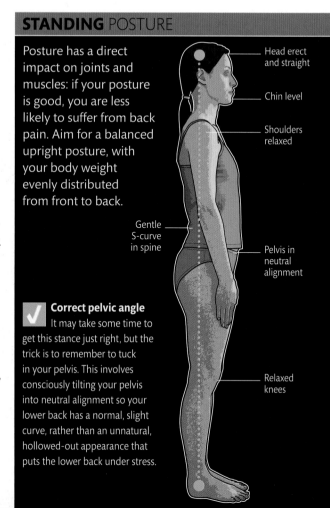

STANDING POSTURE

Posture has a direct impact on joints and muscles: if your posture is good, you are less likely to suffer from back pain. Aim for a balanced upright posture, with your body weight evenly distributed from front to back.

Head erect and straight

Chin level

Shoulders relaxed

Gentle S-curve in spine

Pelvis in neutral alignment

Relaxed knees

✓ **Correct pelvic angle**
It may take some time to get this stance just right, but the trick is to remember to tuck in your pelvis. This involves consciously tilting your pelvis into neutral alignment so your lower back has a normal, slight curve, rather than an unnatural, hollowed-out appearance that puts the lower back under stress.

ORTHOTICS

Orthotics is a branch of medicine that deals with the design, manufacture, and fitting of devices to help support and rectify congenital or acquired problems in your limbs and torso. These orthopedic devices come in various forms, such as back and knee braces, and shoe insoles.

One common problem that can be helped by orthotics is pronation (where your feet roll inward, causing the misalignment of your knee joints and hips). Pronation leads to aches and pains in your lower back where your muscles overcompensate for this weakness. A customized corrective shoe insert may help realign the joints, easing tension and discomfort.

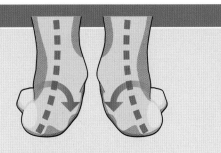

Excessive pronation
Here, the arches of the feet have collapsed, causing the feet to roll inward. This condition results in misalignment of the ligaments, muscles, and tendons in your feet, legs, and back. Left untreated, it can lead to progressive foot and back problems.

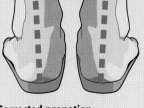

Corrected pronation
Orthotic insoles help correct the misalignment and support your feet properly. They can either be bought over the counter or custom-made.

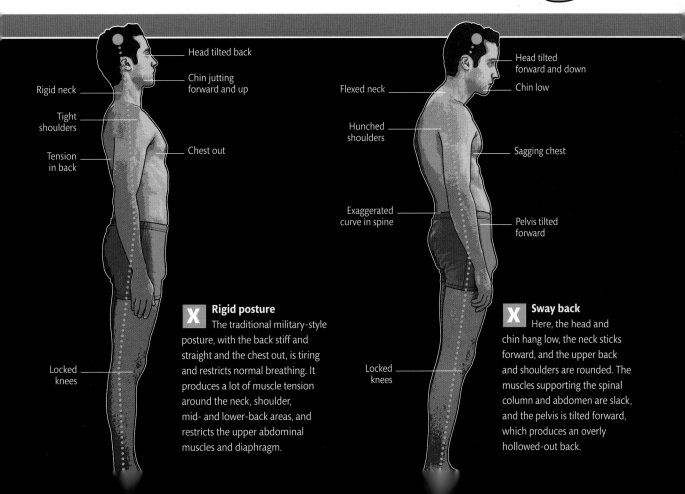

Head tilted back

Chin jutting forward and up

Rigid neck

Tight shoulders

Tension in back

Chest out

Locked knees

X Rigid posture
The traditional military-style posture, with the back stiff and straight and the chest out, is tiring and restricts normal breathing. It produces a lot of muscle tension around the neck, shoulder, mid- and lower-back areas, and restricts the upper abdominal muscles and diaphragm.

Head tilted forward and down

Flexed neck

Chin low

Hunched shoulders

Sagging chest

Exaggerated curve in spine

Pelvis tilted forward

Locked knees

X Sway back
Here, the head and chin hang low, the neck sticks forward, and the upper back and shoulders are rounded. The muscles supporting the spinal column and abdomen are slack, and the pelvis is tilted forward, which produces an overly hollowed-out back.

GOOD SITTING POSTURE

Sitting for prolonged periods of time can trigger pain in your lower back: this is because sitting imposes more strain on your spine than standing or walking. Adopting a correct sitting posture is not difficult and will reduce the stress placed on your back.

RELAXING IN A CHAIR

Good sitting posture does not mean sitting up straight for long periods. You must relax in order to avoid straining your muscles. Anyone attempting to sit bolt upright will gradually slip into a relaxed, slouched position.

When you relax at home, choose a comfortable chair with enough space to let you change your posture: to avoid strained, tense muscles, you must be able to move around while watching television or reading. Cushions placed behind your lower back will help support your spine.

SITTING AT A DESK

Most office workers tend to be desk-bound, which involves sitting at a workstation for most of the day. If you must sit down for long periods of time, use a well-designed chair to reduce the risk of developing either back or neck pain and headaches (**»pp.46–49**), and stretch regularly (**»pp.42–43**).

HEAD AND NECK ALIGNMENT

If, when sitting, you find that your shoulders are rounded or you tend to lean over a desk with your head bent forward, the muscles in your upper back, shoulders, and neck can easily become fatigued. The result can be a painful neck or headaches. Whenever your neck feels tense or you are holding your head forward with your chin out, try to reduce the curve in your neck by pulling your chin back and making the crown of your head the highest point. Neck retraction exercises (**»p.80**) reduce tension by bringing the weight of your head over your spine, so that your neck muscles have less work to do.

SITTING POSTURE

Sitting actually puts more strain on your back than standing, and many of us spend most of our day sitting. That is why it is important to get into good habits early on to help avoid neck and back pain. It is easy to slouch when sitting, so try to catch yourself whenever you do this and make a conscious effort to sit up.

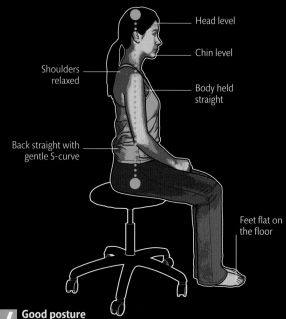

Head level
Chin level
Shoulders relaxed
Body held straight
Back straight with gentle S-curve
Feet flat on the floor

✓ Good posture
Sitting correctly helps keep your bones and joints in correct alignment, and decreases the stress on your spine. Train yourself to be aware of your posture, especially if you have to sit for prolonged

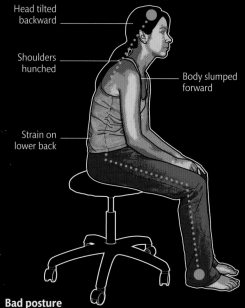

Head tilted backward
Shoulders hunched
Body slumped forward
Strain on lower back

✗ Bad posture
Slouching is one of the most common forms of bad posture. It leads to musculoskeletal pains, backache, joint pains, and tension headaches, and restricts breathing by compressing your diaphragm

PRESSURE ON THE SPINE

These postures show how the pressure within the lumbar disks varies in different positions. Pressures are shown as a percentage relative to standing, which is 100 percent.

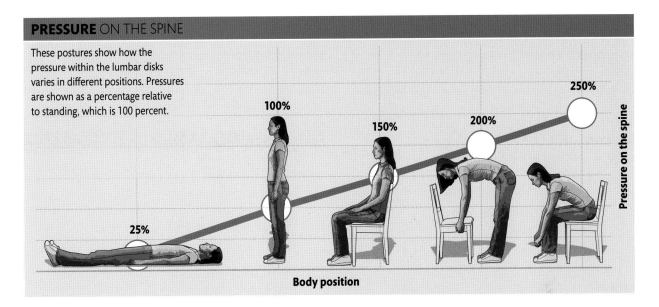

25%

100%

150%

200%

250%

Pressure on the spine

Body position

THE ALEXANDER TECHNIQUE

The Alexander Technique aims to treat and prevent a range of disorders by improving posture. It is based on the principle of relaxing muscles—the neck and shoulder muscles in particular—and of adopting the posture that puts the least amount of stress on your spine.

Actor F. Matthias Alexander developed this technique after progressively and inexplicably losing his voice during performances. He found that, just before delivering a speech on stage, he tended to pull his head backward and down in a manner that cut off his voice. He realized that posture exerts a constant influence on both physiology and psychology.

A qualified Alexander teacher will help you undo any postural habits that have become second nature. She will teach you techniques developed specifically for your own posture, which you should practice every day. The course may last just a few weeks or up to a year.

A course will not cure acute problems such as a disk prolapse or acute facet dysfunction, but can help with "trapped nerves" by making more space. However, once an acute attack is over, the technique helps prevent a recurrence. It is especially useful for avoiding postural pain, and if you are elderly, it may prevent acute episodes of back pain by teaching you to use your back properly.

The technique in practice

Your Alexander teacher will help you eliminate postural defects by studying the way you sit, stand, and move. Your teacher will then tailor the lesson accordingly and may work with you sitting, standing, or lying down, depending on what she feels is required. She will encourage you to imagine that you are being pulled upward from the crown of your head.

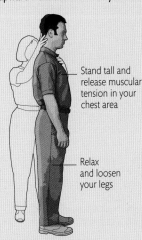

Stand tall and release muscular tension in your chest area

Relax and loosen your legs

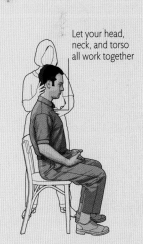

Let your head, neck, and torso all work together

Standing posture

Keep your spine straight when standing, rather than leaning forward and pulling your head back.

Sitting posture

Achieve good sitting posture by encouraging the right amount of curve in your neck, midback, and lower back.

EXERCISE AND SPORT

Exercise is crucial for the health of your back. Working out regularly helps keep your joints supple and strengthens your muscles, allowing your spine to move with ease and comfort.

Research shows that people who are physically fit are healthier and more resistant to back pain and injury. Performing a regular program of stretching and strengthening exercises (**»pp.68–121**) can help improve not only your general fitness levels, but also the strength and mobility of your muscles. Developing good stability and functional movement in the muscles of your abdomen and trunk (your "core") can be particularly useful when it comes to improving your posture. Playing sports regularly offers a range of benefits, helping you improve your fitness, stamina, and endurance levels, lowering your heart rate and blood pressure, burning fat, and reducing stress, all of which can help reduce your chances of back and neck pain.

MOST COMMON CAUSES OF INJURY

The key to avoiding injury is to listen to what your body is telling you and not push yourself too hard. The following factors are the most common causes of sporting injuries:

■ **Failure to warm up**, resulting in your muscles being less responsive and prone to strain.
■ **Overtraining**, which increases the risk of chronic injury by putting continuous pressure on your body.
■ **Excessive loading** on the body, which applies forces to your body tissues for which they are unprepared.
■ **Poor exercise technique**, leading to overloading on body tissues—especially if carried out repeatedly.
■ **Not taking safety precautions**, or ignoring the rules of the sport, so increasing the risk of an accident.
■ **An accident**, often the result of an impact or collision, and usually occurring suddenly.
■ **Inappropriate equipment**, so your body may not be adequately supported or protected from shock.
■ **Recurring injury**, which can weaken your body and make it more susceptible to other injuries.
■ **Genetic factors**, which are intrinsic (belonging to you) and influence the shape and structure of your joints.
■ **Muscle weakness and imbalance**, including poor core stability, which can lead to strains.
■ **Lack of flexibility**, which will decrease your range of motion and limit some of your body's capabilities.
■ **Joint laxity** (a condition which, if you have it, you should already be aware of), which can make it difficult for you to control and stabilize your joints.

WHAT SORT OF EXERCISE SHOULD YOU DO?

The type of exercise you choose depends on your personal needs and preferences. All exercise is good, but to get the most out of your routine, it is advisable to practice a variety of both cardio and low-impact sports. High-impact cardio work, such as skipping and running, can be tough on the joints, especially the knees, so choose low-impact cardio exercises instead. These include walking at a good pace, step aerobics, and using equipment such as kettlebells or dumbbells in your daily exercise workout. Swimming, yoga, and Pilates are low-impact sports, and are ideal for improving the health and suppleness of your back.

CHOOSING THE RIGHT GEAR

Ill-fitting or unsuitable equipment increases the chances of injury. Consider the following tips before buying:
■ Footwear should be suited to your chosen sport and must provide sufficient support and cushioning for your feet and ankles. Seek specialist advice, and always try before you buy.
■ Clothing should be constructed from a material suited to the purpose, such as breathable fabric for warm-weather sports or insulated fabric for cold- and wet-weather sports.
■ Sport-specific equipment, such as bicycles, rackets, and skis, should be custom-fitted to your body's dimensions and weight, and suited to your level of ability.

HOW TO AVOID INJURY

Before doing any exercise, make sure you have the necessary footwear, clothing, and equipment (**»above**). Once you are fully prepared, begin your routine with a 10-minute warm-up (**»opposite**). Warming up helps your body prepare itself for exercise, both mentally and physically, and is the key to unlocking tight muscles. Some people miss out this important part of their routine altogether, but doing so is likely to increase your chances of incurring an injury.

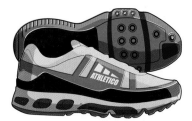

Sports footwear
It is important to buy the right footwear for your chosen sport because there are marked differences in the way various shoes support your feet.

WARM-UP EXERCISES

A good warm-up prepares your body for exercise and reduces the risk of injury. Every warm-up should include the following routines:

■ **Low-impact cardio work** includes exercises that involve your whole body (rather than a specific part of your body); big movements, like going from standing to crouching down and back up again; and ballistic movements, like swinging a kettlebell or a dumbbell. These low-impact, high-intensity exercises will increase your heart rate and blood flow, and warm up your muscles without being tough on your joints. You should begin your warm-up with up to 10 minutes of low-impact cardio work.

■ **Gentle loosening exercises** help loosen up your body if you have been in a sedentary state, and may include rotations of the ankles, hips, wrists, and shoulders, and gentle jogging on the spot. The duration and intensity of the exercises depend on your level of fitness, but should last between 5 and 10 minutes, and produce a light sweat.

■ **Dynamic stretching** contributes to muscular conditioning as well as flexibility. It is best suited to high-level athletes and should only be performed once your body has reached a high degree of flexibility.

■ **Sport-specific exercises** consist of activities and exercises related to your chosen sport, and should be performed at a more vigorous level of exertion than the first stages of your warm-up routine.

Whole body move

Low-impact, high-density moves such as this multijointed squat involve your whole body and work large groups of muscles without pounding the joints.

COOL-DOWN EXERCISES

Cooling down after exercise is as important as warming up. It restores your body to its preexisting state in a controlled manner, helps your body repair itself, and can lessen muscle soreness. Never skip your cool-down, which should consist of the following components:

■ **Gentle walking** allows your heart rate to slow down and recover its resting rate, decreases your body temperature, and aids in the removal of waste products (such as lactic acid) from your muscles. You should spend between 5 and 10 minutes walking after exercise.

■ **Static stretching** involves gradually easing yourself into a stretch position and holding this position. It helps relax your muscles and tendons and allows them to reestablish their normal range of movement. Perform only one or two stretches per muscle group, and hold each position for 20–30 seconds. Take care not to overstretch because this may injure your muscles.

Static stretch

Static stretches should be performed after you have exercised to help your muscles relax. Try to do a selection of both seated and standing stretches to mobilize a whole range of muscles.

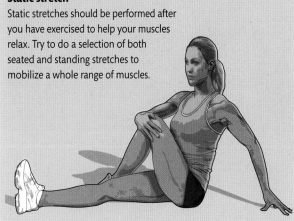

If you have not exercised for a while, make sure you consult your doctor before you start a new regimen. Set yourself clear, realistic goals, and aim to increase the duration and intensity of your exercise routine gradually. You should aim for slow but safe progress.

EXERCISING AFTER INJURY

If you suffer an injury, your body will let you know. Sharp pain is likely to accompany an acute injury, while a dull, nagging pain is usually a sign of the onset of a chronic injury. If you experience pain at any time, modify your activity to reduce strain, and have a period of rest. If the pain recurs, consult your doctor or health care provider.

However, it is important for you to return to an active lifestyle as soon as the worst of the pain is over. Exercising your back is important for recovering from acute backache, and may help those with chronic back pain. After an acute attack, begin exercising as soon as you can move without undue pain. You may ache and feel slightly stiff, but do not let this put you off. Some of the exercises in this book are designed to help with specific back problems, while others are for more general back care (»pp.68–121). Try to exercise once or twice a day, but if this is not possible, practice a few exercises at least once a day. If you are unsure whether you are doing an exercise correctly, seek advice from your physical therapist or a qualified and registered trainer.

THE BENEFITS OF STRETCHING

A gentle stretching routine, when practiced regularly, can help prevent episodes of back pain. Make it part of your daily routine, whether you do any other form of exercise or not.

Stretching increases your range of motion and lengthens and loosens your muscles, making them more flexible and thus helping prevent injury. Simple stretching exercises should be carried out once or twice a day (**»opposite**). These exercises are designed to prevent back pain by increasing movement in your spine and reducing stiffness and pressure on your disks, ligaments, and facet joints. Relax your body and breathe deeply and rhythmically, inhaling before each stretch and exhaling during the movement. Perform the same number of stretches on both sides of your body, and if you feel any pain, stop and come back to it another day.

WHEN TO STRETCH

Ideally, you should aim to stretch daily. If you plan to stretch every day, choose a convenient time and either incorporate the stretches into your regular exercise routine, or just carry them out on their own. Find a time that works best for you, perhaps first thing in the morning or when you get home in the evening. Try to integrate stretching into your day whenever possible: during long periods working at the computer, get into the habit of taking regular stretching breaks; or take 5 minutes to perform a short routine after a flight or a long drive. Even short bursts of stretching can be really invigorating.

PHYSICAL BENEFITS

Incorporating regular stretching into your routine brings many physical benefits, such as:
- Reducing the risk of injury by improving flexibility and balance.
- Helping to balance muscle lengths, which aligns the body, improving and correcting posture.
- Improving flexibility and mobility so that sitting, walking, and standing become easier.
- Promoting relaxation and reducing stress.
- Energizing body and mind.

STRETCHING DURING PREGNANCY

Gentle stretching is generally safe and beneficial during pregnancy and after birth. Relaxin, a hormone produced during pregnancy, relaxes the ligaments in preparation for childbirth, but it may also put you at risk of stretching beyond your normal range. Check with your doctor before you begin stretching.

STRETCHING Q&A

Q | **Why should I follow a stretching program?**
A | We all know that regular exercise is beneficial to our well-being, but if you do not have time for a full workout, then follow the simple stretching program opposite. These exercises are usually performed as a warm-up or cool-down at the start or end of a session, but can also be performed on their own if time is tight. Controlled stretching improves and maintains flexibility and mobility, corrects bad posture, reduces the risk of injury, relieves pain, and even helps counteract the effects of aging.

Q | **Is stretching like yoga or Pilates?**
A | Many people think of yoga or Pilates when they think of stretching. Yoga increases flexibility for the positions of meditation, whereas Pilates concentrates on improving torso strength and control. Stretching is different, in that it aims to align the body, improve posture, and encourage better mechanical movement of the joints, thus reducing wear and tear.

Q | **What happens when I stretch?**
A | Strong muscles, tendons, bones, and ligaments are essential to maintain a healthy body. When you go into a stretch, you feel the pull of your muscles on your bones. Tendons connect muscles to bones, and the pull of stretching helps the tendons remain flexible, preventing injuries. Ligaments connect bone to bone and hold the skeleton together. When stretching, the aim is to elongate the muscles and tendons while protecting the ligaments. Focused stretching aligns the spine and balances the muscle groups that would otherwise become shortened by gravity over time.

Q | **Does everyone benefit from stretching?**
A | Yes. Everyone, both young and old, male or female, and regardless of fitness level, can benefit from stretching. As well as working various muscle groups in the body, stretching energizes the mind, body, and spirit. Stretching consists of simple, straightforward exercises that can be performed almost anywhere.

SIMPLE STRETCHING PROGRAM

This sequence of stretching exercises will work both your upper-back and lower-back muscles (exercises 1–6 and 7–12 respectively). If you spend a lot of time sitting at a desk, the first six exercises will provide a welcome break to your day: do them 5 or 6 times a day. The remaining exercises are for the lower back and should be carried out twice a day, morning and evening.

UPPER BACK

1 Roll-down stretch (》p.84)
Stretches your whole neck and opens up your chest.

▶ 1 set x 3 reps
▶ Hold position for 15 seconds

2 Corner chest stretch (》p.84)
Improves your posture. A great stretch if your chest and shoulders are feeling tight.

▶ 1 set x 3 reps
▶ Hold position for 15 seconds

3 Seated twist stretch (》p.85)
Feel the stretch between and just below your shoulder blades.

▶ 1 set x 3 reps, alternating sides
▶ Hold position for 10 seconds

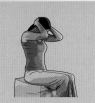

4 Passive neck retraction (》p.80)
Helps you retain a normal range of motion in the neck area.

▶ 1 set x 10 reps
▶ Hold position for 3 seconds

5 Seated back extension (》p.78)
Feel the stretch in your shoulders and upper back.

▶ 1 set x 5 reps
▶ Hold position for 5 seconds

6 Shoulder rotation (》p.69)
Helps mobilize stiff shoulder joints and warms up your trapezius muscles.

▶ 1 set x 10 reps
▶ Slow, flowing movement

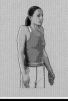

LOWER BACK

7 Standing back extension (》p.110)
Feel instant pain relief in your back as you gently arch backward.

▶ 1 set x 10 reps
▶ Hold position for 3 seconds

8 McKenzie extension (》p.100)
Eases aches in your lower back. An ideal stretch for those who spend most of the day sitting.

▶ 1 set x 10 reps
▶ Hold position for 3 seconds

9 Cat and camel (》p.95)
Lubricates your spine and gets your spinal disks moving.

▶ 1 set x 2 reps
▶ Hold each position for 3 seconds

10 Child's pose (》p.120)
Stretches your spine, hips, thighs, and ankles.

▶ 1 set x 2 reps
▶ Hold position for 20 seconds

11 Lying waist twist (》p.92)
Gives your obliques a good stretch and helps improve core stability.

▶ 1 set x 2 reps, alternating sides
▶ Hold position for 10 seconds

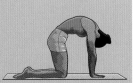

12 Knees-to-chest stretch (》p.110)
Helps ease tight and aching muscles around a strained facet joint.

▶ 1 set x 2 reps
▶ Hold position for 10 seconds

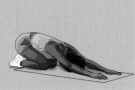
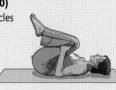
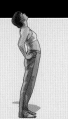

EATING FOR HEALTH

Eating a healthy, balanced diet, and staying hydrated, combined with doing the right exercises at the right intensity and volume, all contribute toward the health of your back.

If you are overweight, you run the risk of putting stress on your spine, so it is a good idea to think about your eating habits and cut down on unhealthy foods. This, coupled with a regular exercise program, will lighten the load on your back.

FOOD, CALORIES, AND BODY WEIGHT

The weight of your body is made up principally of your skeleton, organs, and the muscle, fat, and water that the body carries. Muscular development, body fat, bone density, and the amount of water in the body can all be changed by diet and exercise.

The basic facts about weight gain and loss are simple: you will gain weight if you consume more calories than you burn, and you will lose weight if you eat fewer calories than you need to fuel your basic body functions and lifestyle needs. It is a well-known fact that carrying excess body weight puts a greater strain on your joints, including the joints in your spine, placing them under unnatural pressure and ultimately resulting in back pain.

Some foods contain many calories for a given weight, these are known as energy dense—see Energy Density table (**»below**). Others, such as dietary fiber or roughage, minerals, and vitamins, contain few or no calories, but are still necessary components of your diet.

CALCULATING CALORIES PER FOOD PORTION

Most food products you buy in supermarkets feature a total calorie count per 3½oz (100g) of food. To calculate the calorie intake for the amount of food you actually eat, simply multiply the calorie count for 3½oz by the percentage of ounces (or grams) consumed. For instance, if you eat 5oz (150g) of food, multiply the calorie intake for 3½oz by 150 percent.

ENERGY DENSITY	
Fat	▶ 255 calories per ounce ▶ (9 calories per gram)
Carbohydrate	▶ 113 calories per ounce (4 calories per gram)
Protein	▶ 113 calories per ounce (4 calories per gram)
Water, vitamins, and minerals	Zero calorific value

WHAT IS THE RIGHT LEVEL OF BODY FAT?

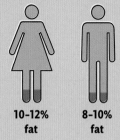

10–12% fat   **8–10% fat**

Athletic
Athletes in training, especially at the elite level, will have significantly less body fat: around 8–10 percent for men and 10–12 percent for women. High levels of fat in relative terms are a serious disadvantage to most athletes, especially in disciplines where "making weight" for a specific competitive class is a priority.

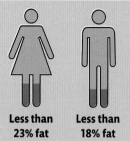

Less than 23% fat   **Less than 18% fat**

Average
It is generally accepted that men should have less than 18 percent of their body weight as fat and women 23 percent or less. A certain amount of body fat is essential for good health. There is plenty of evidence to indicate that carrying less than 5 percent body fat compromises your immune system, making you prone to illness and infections.

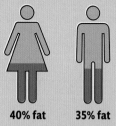

40% fat   **35% fat**

Hazardous
Carrying more fat than the average person is not particularly hazardous to health until you accumulate 35 percent (men) and 40 percent (women) of total body weight as fat. Such levels constitute obesity and have a detrimental effect on health. Too low a level of body fat can also be hazardous, because fat is an important store of energy for aerobic activity.

RECOMMENDED DAILY NUTRIENT INTAKE

There is no universally "correct" balance of daily nutrient intake; the proportions of the main nutrients you need depend on your individual characteristics and lifestyle. However, your food intake should consist, roughly, of:
- 60 percent carbohydrates. These are your main source of energy and are found in fruit and vegetables, bread, pasta, rice, and wholegrain foods.
- 25 percent fat. A good source of energy if consumed in moderation. Unsaturated fat can help lower cholesterol and is found in oily fish, nuts, seeds, and vegetable oils.
- 15 percent protein. Proteins are vital to the growth and repair of muscle and other body tissues. They are found in meat, poultry, fish, eggs, cheese, nuts, and seeds.

YOUR BODY FAT LEVEL

Body Mass Index (BMI) is a measure of whether you are a healthy weight for your height. It is used to determine obesity in both male and female adults and can be calculated using the following equation:

If using imperial measurements:

$$BMI = \left(\frac{\text{weight in pounds}}{\text{height in inches} \times \text{height in inches}} \right) \times 703$$

or, if using metric measurements:

$$BMI = \frac{\text{weight in kilograms}}{\text{height in meters} \times \text{height in meters}}$$

The results should be read as follows:
Underweight: 18.5 or under
Normal: 18.6–24.9
Overweight: 25–29.9
Obese: 30–39.9
Clinically obese: 40 or higher

Although the results are very accurate, BMI does not distinguish between the weight of muscle and that of fat, so that if you are overly muscular (muscle weighs more than fat), the result will not be precise and you will be classified as overweight. So while it is a useful gauge for the general public, BMI needs to be interpreted with caution by anyone with significant muscle mass.

YOUR ENERGY REQUIREMENTS

Your Basic Energy Requirement (BER) is the amount of energy you need to maintain your basic life processes, such as breathing and circulation, when at rest. In addition to your BER, you need energy to live your lifestyle and sustain your personal everyday work and activity patterns. The nature of your job is important: if you do a lot of manual, labor-intensive work, you will have a different energy requirement from someone who leads a more sedentary lifestyle and who works at a desk all day. You can calculate your approximate daily energy requirement by using the table below. The figure you end up with relates to the number of calories you should be consuming per day to retain your present body weight.

CALCULATING YOUR ENERGY REQUIREMENTS

Locate your age range and enter your weight into the appropriate equation to find your BER. Then, multiply this figure by the factor associated with your type of lifestyle—sedentary, moderately active, or very active. The figure you arrive at is the level of calorie intake that will allow you to maintain your present body weight. If you take in more calories than your daily energy requirement (including the exercise you get), you will gain weight. If you take in fewer calories than your daily energy requirement (including exercise), you will lose weight.

Male		
▶ 10–17 years	▶ 8 x weight in lb ▶ 17.5 x weight in kg	▶ + 651
▶ 18–29 years	▶ 7 x weight in lb ▶ 15.3 x weight in kg	▶ + 679
▶ 30–59 years	▶ 5.2 x weight in lb ▶ 11.6 x weight in kg	▶ + 879
▶ 60+ years	▶ 6 x weight in lb ▶ 13.5 x weight in kg	▶ + 487
Female		
▶ 10–17 years	▶ 5.5 x weight in lb ▶ 12.2 x weight in kg	▶ + 746
▶ 18–29 years	▶ 6.7 x weight in lb ▶ 14.7 x weight in kg	▶ + 496
▶ 30–59 years	▶ 3.9 x weight in lb ▶ 8.7 x weight in kg	▶ + 829
▶ 60+ years	▶ 4.7 x weight in lb ▶ 10.5 x weight in kg	▶ + 596

Sedentary multiply by 1.5
Moderately active multiply by 1.6
Very active multiply by 1.7

AT THE OFFICE

If your work involves sitting at a computer day after day, it is important to set up your work station correctly to give your back maximum support. Maintaining good posture is essential to protect your back, neck, and shoulders, and to avoid muscle tension and headaches.

Sitting imposes more strain on the spine than standing or walking, so a well-designed chair is very important if you spend long hours at a desk. If you are prone to lower-back pain, make sure that your chair is at the correct height for your leg length—your feet should be flat on the floor. Keep your seat horizontal, and sit close enough to the desk so that you can use your keyboard without having to stretch your arms out. To avoid tension in your shoulders and neck, the height of the desk should allow you to touch the keyboard with your fingers while keeping your arms bent just slightly below the horizontal. Rest your arms on the desk, keeping them parallel to the floor, but avoid leaning on them. You should change position regularly and take breaks away from your desk.

HEAD AND NECK ALIGNMENT

If you spend time leaning over a desk with your back rounded and your head bent forward, the muscles in your upper back, shoulders, and neck are likely to become fatigued.

SITTING IN AN ERGONOMIC CHAIR

Adjust the height of your chair so that your feet are flat on the floor, and tilt the back slightly downward to support you when you lean forward to work. Ideally, the chair should also tilt backward so that you can relax. The seat should be angled so that your hips are slightly higher than your knees.

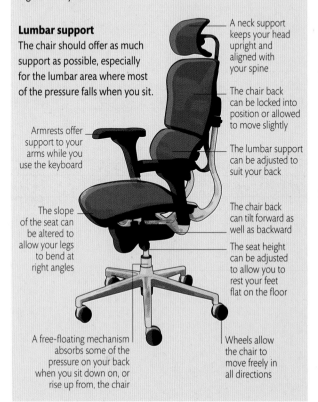

Lumbar support
The chair should offer as much support as possible, especially for the lumbar area where most of the pressure falls when you sit.

A neck support keeps your head upright and aligned with your spine

The chair back can be locked into position or allowed to move slightly

The lumbar support can be adjusted to suit your back

Armrests offer support to your arms while you use the keyboard

The chair back can tilt forward as well as backward

The slope of the seat can be altered to allow your legs to bend at right angles

The seat height can be adjusted to allow you to rest your feet flat on the floor

A free-floating mechanism absorbs some of the pressure on your back when you sit down on, or rise up from, the chair

Wheels allow the chair to move freely in all directions

WORKING ON A DESKTOP COMPUTER

Even when you have set up your workspace so that the desk, chair, keyboard, and monitor are in the right place for you, you still need to be conscious of your posture. Good posture will ensure your back is supported and your spine aligned. It will help prevent backache as well as shoulder and neck pain that can lead to headaches.

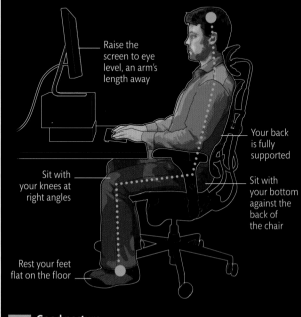

Raise the screen to eye level, an arm's length away

Your back is fully supported

Sit with your knees at right angles

Sit with your bottom against the back of the chair

Rest your feet flat on the floor

✓ Good posture
With your spine supported by an ergonomic chair, your back, shoulders, and neck are aligned. Your body appears alert and ready to work but at the same time it is relaxed with no areas of tension.

The result can be a painful neck or headaches. Chronic neck tension can also cause migraines. Whenever your neck feels tense or you are holding your head forward with your chin out, reduce the curve in your neck by pulling your chin back and making the crown of your head the highest point. Neck retraction exercises (**»p.80**) reduce tension by bringing the weight of your head more directly over your spine, so that your neck muscles have less work to do.

UNDER THE DESK

Keep your feet flat on the floor and your knees slightly below your hips. Ensure that there is adequate space from the back of your knees to the edge of the chair—roughly the width of three fingers—to allow your legs to move freely. Avoid crossing your legs as this results in a poor hip position.

USING A COMPUTER

The following simple rules will help you avoid some of the common problems associated with working at a computer:
- Place your monitor and keyboard directly in front of you.
- Use a support to keep your hands and wrists aligned.
- Set up your monitor so that the screen is an arm's length away from you and the toolbars at the top are at eye level.
- Use a hard-copy holder to avoid constantly looking down.
- Instead of leaning toward the screen in order to read the type, zoom in to enlarge the text—and have your eyes tested.
- Keep the mouse near but with space to move it freely.
- Touch the keys lightly and touch type if you can, to avoid having to look down at the keys.
- Keep your elbows vertically under your shoulders and close to the sides of your body, or on an armrest.

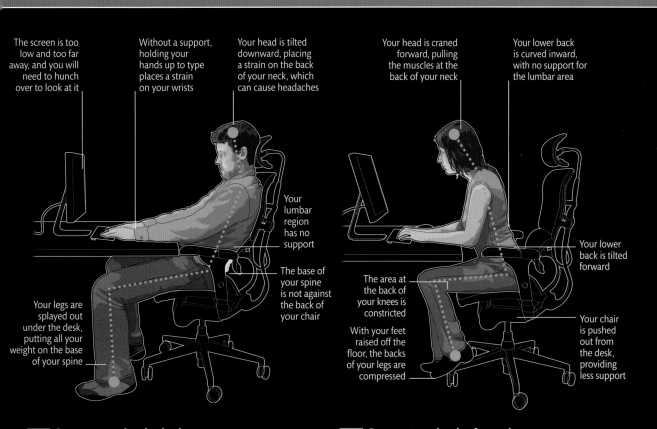

The screen is too low and too far away, and you will need to hunch over to look at it

Without a support, holding your hands up to type places a strain on your wrists

Your head is tilted downward, placing a strain on the back of your neck, which can cause headaches

Your lumbar region has no support

The base of your spine is not against the back of your chair

Your legs are splayed out under the desk, putting all your weight on the base of your spine

Your head is craned forward, pulling the muscles at the back of your neck

Your lower back is curved inward, with no support for the lumbar area

Your lower back is tilted forward

Your chair is pushed out from the desk, providing less support

The area at the back of your knees is constricted

With your feet raised off the floor, the backs of your legs are compressed

X Poor posture–leaning back
It is very easy to slump when you have been working at your desk for hours at a stretch. Here, the shoulders are rounded inward and the head is leaning forward, both of which can lead to upper-back pain.

X Poor posture–leaning forward
Leaning into the monitor means that your neck and upper back have no support, and your legs are constricted. The lumbar area is also unsupported and your knees are strained.

USING A LAPTOP

Many people spend time using a laptop at home, but since laptops are designed to be portable and lightweight rather than adjustable, this can easily lead to back problems. It is common to use them while lying on the sofa or slumped with your back and neck in an awkward position. However, if you are spending hours working on a laptop, you need to take care to set up a healthy working environment, applying the same principles as you would to arranging your workstation in the office.

You will need a supportive office chair—ideally an ergonomic one that can be adjusted—and a desk or table that is the right height for you. Follow the advice given for sitting at an office desk (**»pp.46–47**) and avoid leaning forward over the laptop. You should also take care not to slump at the shoulders or crane your neck, since both of these positions will lead to tension in your neck and shoulders, and pain in your upper back.

Laptop set-up

If you position your laptop so that the screen is at the right height, then the keyboard will not be, and vice versa. The screen should be an arm's length away from you and at eye level, while your arms should be resting at right angles to your body when using the keyboard. If you need to work on your laptop for any length of time, a separate keyboard and mouse are easier to use and adjust to your needs, or you may wish to invest in a separate desktop computer.

USING LAPTOPS AND OTHER PORTABLE DEVICES

Laptops, netbooks, and tablets are compact and easy to carry around but you cannot adjust them to make them comfortable to work on for long periods. You risk back problems if you use these devices without taking measures to ensure that you maintain good posture.

Ideally, you should set up at a desk, using a purpose-made stand—or a box, or books—to raise the device to the correct level, and a separate keyboard and mouse. Even when working away from your desk there are steps that you can take to protect yourself from injury.

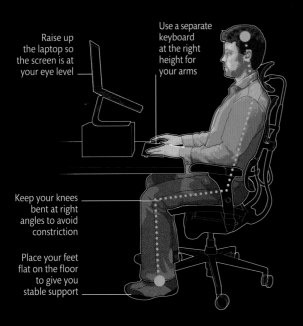

Raise up the laptop so the screen is at your eye level

Use a separate keyboard at the right height for your arms

Keep your knees bent at right angles to avoid constriction

Place your feet flat on the floor to give you stable support

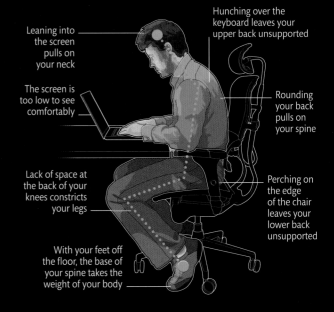

Hunching over the keyboard leaves your upper back unsupported

Leaning into the screen pulls on your neck

The screen is too low to see comfortably

Rounding your back pulls on your spine

Lack of space at the back of your knees constricts your legs

Perching on the edge of the chair leaves your lower back unsupported

With your feet off the floor, the base of your spine takes the weight of your body

✓ Good posture
Keep your head and neck aligned and your back straight. Face forward and keep your arms bent at right angles at the elbow when using the keyboard. Make sure your spine is supported by keeping your back against the back of the chair.

✗ Bad posture
Without a laptop stand and separate mouse and keyboard it is difficult to sit upright while using a laptop. Your head cranes downward and brings your neck and shoulders with it. Working on the keyboard can feel cramped, pulling on your shoulders and upper back.

Laptop stands are useful for raising your laptop to the correct height. Some of these are designed to be used when you are out, while others might form part of a more permanent set-up in your home—it is worth spending time finding out which stand works best for you.

Using a laptop on the sofa

Of course, some of the time spent on your laptop will be for pleasure rather than work, but you still need to protect your back. Laptop cushions provide a comfortable and stable base for your machine and make it easier to use while sitting upright on a sofa. Keep your feet flat on the floor and your back against the back of the sofa. Use cushions to support your back, if needed.

USING A PHONE

If you make and receive phone calls while working at your computer, it is tempting to hold the handset between your shoulder and ear while you continue to work. However, gripping the phone with your shoulder can cause tension in your shoulder, neck, and upper back. Follow the suggestions below to avoid these problems:

■ Wear a headset rather than using a handset: this keeps your hands free so you can continue working.
■ Sit facing your desk and keyboard while you talk—twisting around places unnecessary stress on your back.
■ Keep the keyboard within easy reach so that your arms and shoulders stay relaxed. Avoid overreaching.

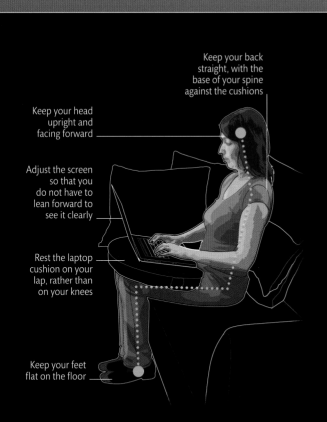

Keep your head upright and facing forward

Keep your back straight, with the base of your spine against the cushions

Adjust the screen so that you do not have to lean forward to see it clearly

Rest the laptop cushion on your lap, rather than on your knees

Keep your feet flat on the floor

✓ **Using a laptop away from your desk**
While it is best to work at a desk, if you have to sit on a couch, use cushions to support your back and a laptop cushion to steady your machine. Sit upright with the laptop in front of you and your elbows under your shoulders. Avoid leaning forward or to the side.

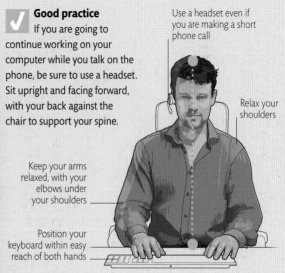

✓ **Good practice**
If you are going to continue working on your computer while you talk on the phone, be sure to use a headset. Sit upright and facing forward, with your back against the chair to support your spine.

Use a headset even if you are making a short phone call

Relax your shoulders

Keep your arms relaxed, with your elbows under your shoulders

Position your keyboard within easy reach of both hands

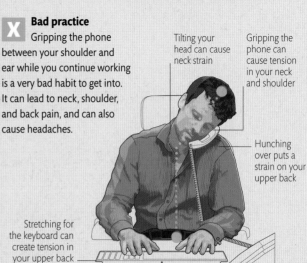

✗ **Bad practice**
Gripping the phone between your shoulder and ear while you continue working is a very bad habit to get into. It can lead to neck, shoulder, and back pain, and can also cause headaches.

Tilting your head can cause neck strain

Gripping the phone can cause tension in your neck and shoulder

Hunching over puts a strain on your upper back

Stretching for the keyboard can create tension in your upper back

LIFTING AND CARRYING

When lifting a load, it is common to round your back and take the weight on your spine. It is much safer to keep your back straight and let your more powerful abdominal and leg muscles do the work instead.

It puts strain on your spine if you round your back forward or arch your back and stick your hips out when lifting. Both positions shift the weight down onto your lower back, which can lead to backache. Instead, you should straighten your back against the pull of the load, keep your hips in a flexed position, and use your leg muscles to take the strain.

If you are carrying something in front of you, take care not to increase the arch in your lower back or to lean backward, and avoid pushing your hips forward. Your abdominal and back muscles should support your back,

while your leg muscles take the weight. If you are carrying something on your back, try to avoid leaning forward to take the strain, as this places the weight on your curved spine rather than your muscles.

In general, keep your back straight and avoid lifting anything that is too heavy for you. As well as getting into the habit of using the muscles in your abdomen and legs, check your posture in the mirror to find out how your spine feels when it is straight and when your pelvis is in a neutral position.

WARNING!

Don't try to lift something that is too heavy for you because this could strain your back. If you are not sure of the weight, make an assessment by following steps 1 and 2 below, but just lifting the box a little way off the ground. If it is too heavy, get help to lift it.

LIFTING A BOX

Before you lift a box, take a moment to assess how heavy it is. Squat down, keeping your back straight and using your leg muscles to lift the weight; come up smoothly. Keep the load close to your body when you lift and carry it.

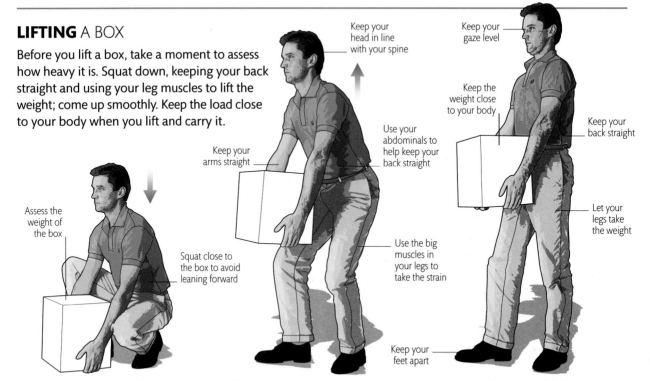

Keep your head in line with your spine

Keep your gaze level

Keep the weight close to your body

Use your abdominals to help keep your back straight

Keep your back straight

Keep your arms straight

Assess the weight of the box

Let your legs take the weight

Squat close to the box to avoid leaning forward

Use the big muscles in your legs to take the strain

Keep your feet apart

1 Squat down on your haunches with the box between your legs and one foot on either side. Try to assess whether the box is too large, heavy, or awkwardly shaped before you attempt to lift it.

2 Keeping your back straight, slide your hands under the box and grasp it on either side. Stand up in one smooth motion, keeping the object close to you.

3 Do not bend your back, and be careful not to lean backward; use your abdominal muscles to support your spine. Keep your weight equal on both legs.

CARRYING BAGS

When you are packing shopping, distribute the items between several bags to balance the weight, then spread the load so that you are carrying an equal weight in each hand. When carrying a single heavier item, such as a laptop or file, a bag that you can wear across your body or a backpack is a good idea. Choose one with a wide strap and keep the weight close to your body. Remember to swap the bag from one shoulder to the other occasionally. Take care when putting them on and taking them off—use a table as a halfway point.

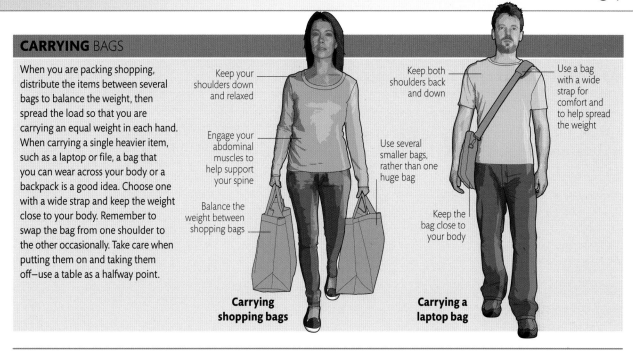

Keep your shoulders down and relaxed

Engage your abdominal muscles to help support your spine

Balance the weight between shopping bags

Carrying shopping bags

Keep both shoulders back and down

Use several smaller bags, rather than one huge bag

Keep the bag close to your body

Use a bag with a wide strap for comfort and to help spread the weight

Carrying a laptop bag

LIFTING A LONG LOAD

When you need to lift a longer load, begin by making an assessment of the weight and, if you can't get someone else to carry the other end, assess whether it is safe for you to lift on your own. If it is, squat down with your legs astride one end of the load. You can either keep your legs in line or put one in front of the other. Try not to lean forward, and keep your back straight throughout.

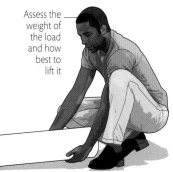

Assess the weight of the load and how best to lift it

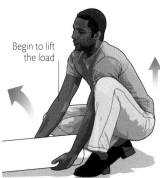

Begin to lift the load

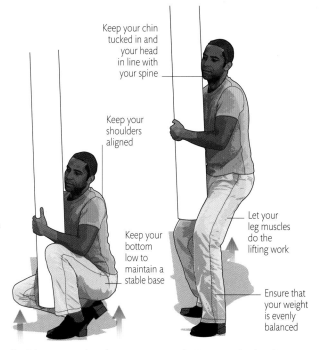

Keep your chin tucked in and your head in line with your spine

Keep your shoulders aligned

Keep your bottom low to maintain a stable base

Let your leg muscles do the lifting work

Ensure that your weight is evenly balanced

1 Squat down with one end of the load between your feet. Slide both hands underneath the load and take a firm grip.

2 Raise the end nearest to you, tilting it away from your body until the load is balanced upright on the other end. Step forward if necessary.

3 Move your hand underneath the end of the load and bring it close to your body, resting the load against your shoulder.

4 Keeping the load vertical and, gripping it firmly, stand up slowly, keeping your back straight throughout.

DOING HOUSEWORK

Many household chores involve bending and lifting. You can reduce the strain on your back by learning new techniques and using different ways to approach your tasks.

As a general rule of thumb, if some chores are causing you pain, vary your activity, rest frequently, and avoid too many repetitive movements.

In the kitchen, be aware of your posture when you are preparing food on the kitchen counter. Ideally, the counter should be slightly lower than your elbow. Stand close to it to avoid overreaching, and keep your back straight. It may feel more comfortable to have one foot in front of the other, or one foot resting on a small step or on the base of the cabinet. The sink should also be at elbow height, so you are not forced to stoop when washing up. If necessary, put a washing-up bowl on the worktop or on top of another bowl to get it to the right height.

To reach into high cabinets, you may find it useful to keep a low stepstool in the kitchen. Take things down individually, and avoid overstretching so that you do not lose your balance. You may need to rearrange the contents of your cabinets to store the most-used items on the lowest shelves. Keep your back straight when you bend to the oven or dishwasher.

WORKING AROUND THE HOME

Approaching everyday chores in a different way can help protect your back from strain. Prepare the area in advance so you have everything you need in position, and work slowly to avoid sudden twists or jolts to your back.

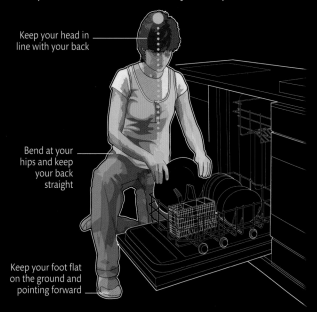

Keep your head in line with your back

Bend at your hips and keep your back straight

Keep your foot flat on the ground and pointing forward

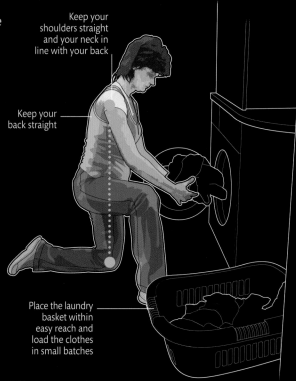

Keep your shoulders straight and your neck in line with your back

Keep your back straight

Place the laundry basket within easy reach and load the clothes in small batches

☑ Loading the dishwasher
Pile up your dirty dishes beside the dishwasher within easy reach. Kneel down on one knee, and keep your other leg perpendicular. Keeping your back straight, put the items in one by one, and avoid leaning too far forward and overreaching. Use your leg muscles to take the strain. An alternative method is to squat down beside the machine with your legs apart and your knees in line with your ankles.

☑ Using a washing machine
If you have a front-loading washing machine, squat, sit, or put one knee on the floor while you fill or empty it. If you have a top-loading machine, avoid bending and twisting as much as possible by keeping your basket at the same height as the machine. Reach into the machine with one arm and raise the opposite leg for balance.

CLEANING THE FLOOR

Stand facing the area you are cleaning, and try not to twist or reach too far forward. Move the broom, mop, or vacuum cleaner and your body at the same time. If you are using an upright vacuum cleaner, keep it close to your body. Stand with one foot in front of the other with your knees bent, and, rather than bending, rock backward and forward. Avoid dragging the vacuum cleaner, and instead make short movements backward and forward. If you are using a cylinder vacuum cleaner, keep the hose fully extended. To clean under a table, bend at your hips and knees, keeping your back as straight as you can. When it comes to buying a new cleaner, choose a high-powered lightweight model with a long hose and a wide nozzle.

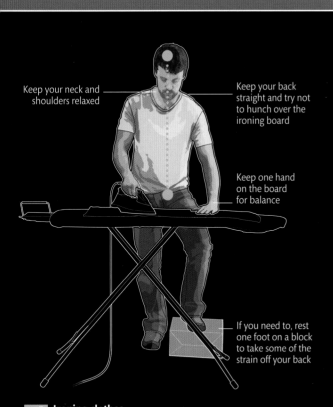

Keep your neck and shoulders relaxed

Keep your back straight and try not to hunch over the ironing board

Keep one hand on the board for balance

If you need to, rest one foot on a block to take some of the strain off your back

✓ Ironing clothes

Raise the ironing board up to around hip height to avoid stooping. You should be able to move your arms freely without having to lift your shoulders. Stand close to the board, and, with one foot facing forward and the other in the direction the board is pointing, sway from one foot to the other as you iron. Alternatively, you can take the weight off your legs by perching on the side of an armchair or sofa while you iron.

HOUSEWORK Q&A

Q | **What should I wear?**

A | Wear comfortable clothing so you can move around freely. Put on old clothes so you don't have to worry about them getting dirty or wet.

Q | **How should I reach for things in the refrigerator?**

A | When organizing your refrigerator, keep the items that you use regularly on the middle shelf to avoid having to do too much reaching and stretching. When you do have to bend, squat down or place one knee on the floor, and use the power in your legs to get up. When buying a new refrigerator, if space allows, choose one that sits above the freezer, rather than below it.

Q | **What is the best way to make a bed?**

A | Squat down or kneel by the bed when you tuck in the sheets. Buy fitted sheets and comforters to make it easier. Fit smooth-running casters if you need to move the bed.

Q | **How should I approach general cleaning tasks?**

A | Use long-handled implements to avoid overstretching. If necessary, kneel down to clean.

Q | **How can I make doing the laundry easier?**

A | Place the laundry basket on a stool nearby to avoid having to bend down to the floor. Small items can be placed in a mesh bag so that they are easier to get hold of. Wet laundry will be much heavier to deal with, so you may want to take it out of the washer one piece at a time. Keep the clothesline at a sensible height so you don't have to strain to reach it.

Q | **If I suffer from ongoing back pain, how can I make household chores easier for myself?**

A | Consider making small adaptations to your home environment. For example, an ergonomically-designed kitchen may make cooking much easier.

Q | **How should I approach DIY?**

A | Don't twist your trunk when doing any lifting. Let other parts of your body, such as shoulders, pelvis, or thighs, take the weight. Don't overstretch. Avoid unnecessary effort—buy any tools that will make the task easier.

Q | **What if there are some chores I just cannot do?**

A | Ask friends and family for help, and consider paying a professional to do the more strenuous tasks for you.

WORKING IN YOUR GARDEN

Many garden tasks involve crouching, bending, and lifting. You can minimize the strain on your back by working in an upright position, following the rules for lifting (»pp.50–51), and varying the tasks to reduce the strain on your back.

When lifting and carrying, use the strength in your legs rather than your back to move the weight. If you are performing any work that is high up, such as pruning trees or fixing fences, use a stepladder and long-handled tools so that you are not forced to overstretch. When mowing, face in the direction you are moving, engage your abdominal muscles, keep your back straight, and hold your head up. If you are weeding or planting, kneel down on a cushioned pad or sit on a low stool. If your back is very bad, you may want to convert your garden to raised beds, or grow plants in a greenhouse instead.

WARNING!

Approach your activities in the garden as you would any form of exercise. Wear suitable clothing, perform simple stretching exercises to warm up beforehand, take regular breaks, and drink plenty of water. If necessary, ask someone to help.

DIGGING IN THE GARDEN

This is a task that will put pressure on your back, whether you usually suffer from back pain or not. The key is to avoid lifting too much soil in one load. Work at a steady pace, and if you feel any twinges, rest before resuming. There are specially adapted spades available that have levers to make the task of digging and turning soil easier.

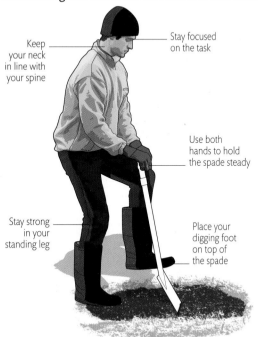

Keep your neck in line with your spine

Stay focused on the task

Use both hands to hold the spade steady

Stay strong in your standing leg

Place your digging foot on top of the spade

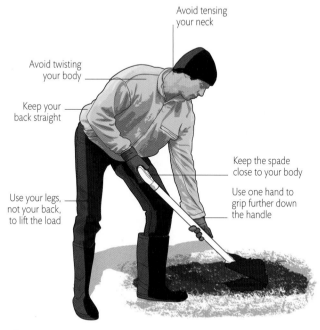

Avoid tensing your neck

Avoid twisting your body

Keep your back straight

Keep the spade close to your body

Use your legs, not your back, to lift the load

Use one hand to grip further down the handle

1 Keeping your back straight, push the spade into the ground using your body weight, rather than your muscle power. Bend at your knees and hips rather than your waist, and do not grip the spade too tightly. Before you start to lift the soil, cut around the sides of each spadeful.

2 Hold the handle at the end and use the spade as a lever to ease the soil out. Raise the soil using the handle of the spade near its base for leverage. Move your feet and turn toward where you want to place the load: do not stand in one position and twist your back.

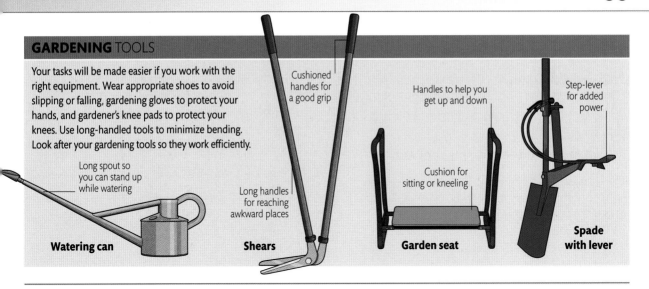

GARDENING TOOLS

Your tasks will be made easier if you work with the right equipment. Wear appropriate shoes to avoid slipping or falling, gardening gloves to protect your hands, and gardener's knee pads to protect your knees. Use long-handled tools to minimize bending. Look after your gardening tools so they work efficiently.

Cushioned handles for a good grip

Handles to help you get up and down

Step-lever for added power

Long spout so you can stand up while watering

Long handles for reaching awkward places

Cushion for sitting or kneeling

Watering can

Shears

Garden seat

Spade with lever

SHOVELING EARTH

Much of the advice for digging also applies to shoveling—the difference being that you crouch down low, and move the spade with a more shallow movement. In general, and where possible, you should wait for the right conditions: try to avoid digging or shoveling when the soil is wet and heavy or dry and compacted, as this will make your task more arduous and could place more strain on your back.

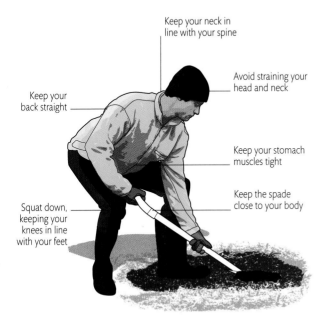

Keep your neck in line with your spine

Avoid straining your head and neck

Keep your back straight

Keep your stomach muscles tight

Keep the spade close to your body

Squat down, keeping your knees in line with your feet

Avoid making any sudden movements with your neck

Keep your shoulders back and down

Hold your head up

Try to avoid hunching forward

Avoid turning your upper body; move your arms to shift the soil

Lever the spade up against your thigh

Squat down low to the ground

1 Squat down, bending at the knees and hips and keeping your back as straight as possible. Lean forward but maintain a low, stable center of gravity. Slide the shovel along the ground, resting the back of your top hand against the inside of your knee or thigh to use as a lever.

2 Squat down to the ground and push the spade forward in one smooth movement. When your spade is full, throw the soil to one side using a sideways movement, rather than lifting it. Do your best to move your arms but minimize the movement of your upper body.

DRIVING YOUR CAR

It can be agonizing to drive your car if you suffer from a bad back or neck problems, unless your car is equipped with a good car seat and well-placed controls.

Even if you do not usually suffer from back or neck pain, driving is one of the activities that can encourage these problems, because you are not only subject to constant vibrations and sudden movements, but are often forced to sit in one position for a long time. Therefore you need to sit in a position that keeps your arms and legs relaxed and that provides proper support for your body, especially your back. Before driving off, always make sure that you are demonstrating good posture: adjust the height of your seat, the angle of the backrest, and the distance from the steering wheel. You should be able to look into your rear view and side mirrors comfortably without straining your neck.

IN THE DRIVER'S SEAT

Try to get into the habit of relaxing your neck and shoulder muscles while you are driving. It is helpful to become aware of times when you grip the wheel too tightly or hold it too high up with your arms outstretched. If your shoulders are hunching up toward your ears, develop a relaxed and steady breathing rhythm, and with each breath let go of the tightness in your muscles, slowly dropping your shoulders. Gently work your head and neck back into a more relaxed position against your headrest.

It is also advisable to take frequent breaks when making long trips. Stop the car and walk around for a few minutes, perform some simple stretches, and roll your shoulders with small circular movements.

If you are buying a new car, look at the car seat design very closely; make sure that the seats are adjustable, and take a test drive to see whether you find them comfortable.

GETTING OUT OF A CAR

Getting out of a car is usually harder than getting in, because your body may be stiff and immobile from the trip. To get into a car, simply reverse the process outlined below; the difference being that you turn away

from the car and support yourself by holding onto the door, bend your knees, and lower your bottom onto the car seat. Once you are seated, shift your right leg and then your left leg carefully into the car.

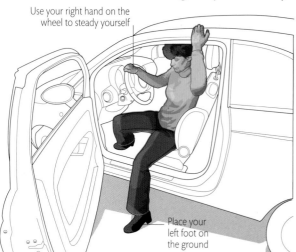

Use your right hand on the wheel to steady yourself

Place your left foot on the ground

1 Park away from the curb and move the car seat back to give yourself plenty of room. Open the door, and, holding onto the wheel with one hand and the car roof with the other, use them as leverage, turning your body toward the door.

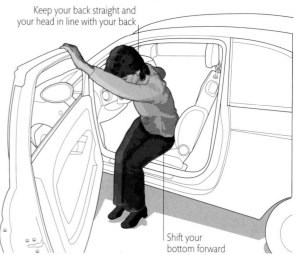

Keep your back straight and your head in line with your back

Shift your bottom forward

2 Place your right foot on the ground next to your left foot. Once you are facing the door, shift your bottom forward to the edge of the seat and place your left hand on the upper frame of the door. Keep your right hand on the steering wheel.

CORRECT DRIVING POSITION

To avoid subjecting yourself to unnecessary strain when driving, work through this checklist next time you sit in your car:

■ **Make sure that** the cushioning of the car seat does not slope toward the middle, or too much weight will be borne by your pelvic bones instead of your thighs. The seat must be firm enough to resist the indirect forces you experience when using the pedals; however, if the seat is too hard, the engine vibrations will be transmitted up your spine.

■ **Check that the backrest** gives good support to your lower back. Ideally, your car should have built-in lumbar support; if not, use a rolled-up towel, or cushions that can be attached by a strap. If you can, alter the angle of the backrest to an optimum of between five and ten degrees behind the vertical.

■ **Rest your head** on the headrest, relaxing your neck and shoulders while looking straight ahead. The headrest should be slightly padded, and adjustable both up and down, forward and back. The top of the headrest should be at least level with your forehead in order to effectively reduce whiplash strain.

■ **Make sure your feet** rest comfortably on the pedals. Check that the pedals are not too stiff (especially the clutch), too high off the floor, or set too far to one side.

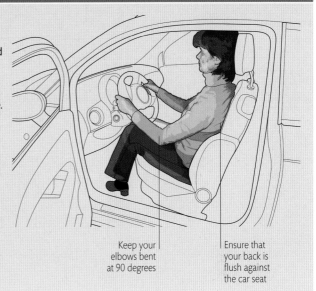

Keep your elbows bent at 90 degrees

Ensure that your back is flush against the car seat

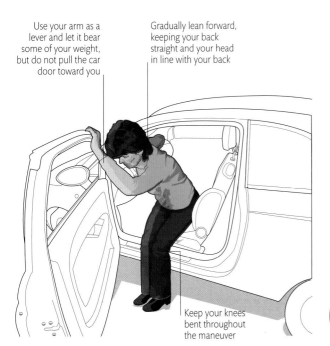

Use your arm as a lever and let it bear some of your weight, but do not pull the car door toward you

Gradually lean forward, keeping your back straight and your head in line with your back

Keep your knees bent throughout the maneuver

3 Start to lean out of the car, using your outstretched arm to help control the movement. Keep your head lifted and your knees bent throughout; use your hips to move, rather than your lower back.

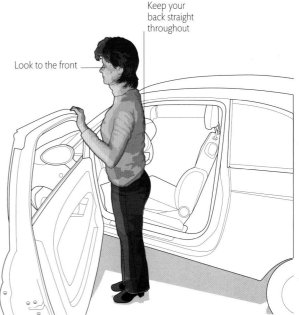

Keep your back straight throughout

Look to the front

4 Bearing the weight in your legs rather than your back, gradually straighten from the knees until you are standing. While this procedure may take a little longer than usual, it is worth getting into the habit of exiting a car in this way.

LYING DOWN AND SLEEPING

You may find that you are most comfortable when you are lying down. This is because a lying position relieves most of the pressure that your body weight puts on your spine. You don't have to lie flat on your back, however: try out the positions shown below until you find one that works best for you.

YOUR BED

If you find that your back pain is at its worst in the morning or that this is the only time your back aches, you may need a new mattress. Likewise, if you have only developed pain since you bought a new mattress, you should consider replacing it. Bear in mind that aching and stiffness can also result from inactivity, so it may not matter which surface you lie on.

When purchasing a mattress, make sure you choose one that is firm, finely sprung, and provides sufficient support, and is at least 6 in (15 cm) longer than you are to allow freedom of movement. No matter how good your mattress is, a sagging bed base can harm your back, so make sure that the base is firm and strong enough to support your mattress.

Adjustable beds are now widely available and affordable, and offer positional comfort. They allow you to raise your legs or head to any angle at the touch of a button, meaning that you can even set them for the Fowler position (**»below**).

POSITIONS TO LIE IN

Lying on your front increases the curve in your lower back, which aggravates backache caused by facet joint problems. However, such a position will probably not hurt your back if your pain is caused by a herniated disk.

SLEEPING POSITIONS

If you suffer from back pain there are a number of positions you can adopt to help you sleep. Different types of pillows or a folded towel can alleviate back pain. Try these positions and see what works for you.

Use a McKenzie night roll (a specially designed cushion) to support your waist

Place a small pillow between your knees to support your hips

Place a body pillow between your legs for support

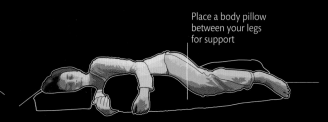

Lying on your side I
Lie on your side with a pillow supporting your head and a McKenzie night roll supporting your waist so your spine is straight. Place a pillow between your knees to help with your alignment.

Lying on your side II
Rest your head on a support pillow (**»opposite**) so that your head is in line with your spine and use a body pillow to support your entire body. Pregnant women will find this type of pillow particularly comfortable.

Rest your head on a neck support pillow

Keep your spine aligned

Use a folded towel under your knees to support your hips

Bend your knees at right angles and rest your legs on a few pillows

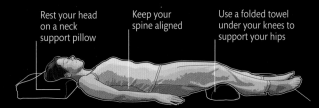

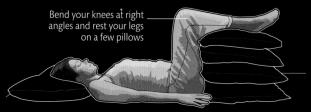

Lying on your back
Lie on your back and rest your head on a neck support pillow to prevent your head flopping from side to side. Place a rolled-up towel under your knees to help with lower-back pain.

The Fowler position
If lying flat on your back causes you pain, lie with your knees bent at right angles and your calves supported on a stack of pillows. This reduces the curve in your lower back and minimizes the pressure on your disks.

Lying flat on your back with your legs straight may also increase the curve in your lower back and cause backache. The Fowler position (**»opposite**) helps flatten out this excessive curve and relaxes the psoas muscles, which run from your lower back to your thighs. If you have acute back pain, you should place several pillows under your knees, but for most other conditions, a rolled-up towel may be enough.

With an adjustable bed (**»opposite**), you can raise or lower your head and legs to relieve aching limbs, or lie in a semirecumbent position if you have breathing or cardiac problems. The bed may also have a vibration mode to micromassage your joints.

To avoid neck pain, make sure your head rests fairly square on your shoulders to minimize the strain. You should only use one pillow if you lie on your back; if you sleep on your side, the width of your shoulders will determine whether you need one or two pillows to support your head.

PILLOW SUPPORT

It is important to ensure you get the correct support from your pillow. To test a pillow, lift it horizontally, with the edge of your hand running across the center: if it stays more or less level, it is fine; if it sags, you should replace it. If you wake with a stiff neck, try twisting the pillow into a butterfly shape or use a rolled towel placed around your neck to act as a soft collar. Alternatively, try a neck support pillow, which supports your neck and prevents your head lolling from side to side.

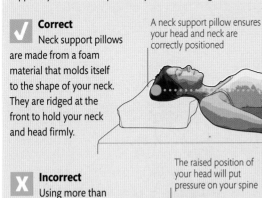

✓ Correct
Neck support pillows are made from a foam material that molds itself to the shape of your neck. They are ridged at the front to hold your neck and head firmly.

A neck support pillow ensures your head and neck are correctly positioned

✗ Incorrect
Using more than one pillow can cause excessive flexion of your head and neck, which can put pressure on your spine and cause or exacerbate pain.

The raised position of your head will put pressure on your spine

SEX AND BACK PAIN Q&A

Q | Can I still have sex if I have back pain?

A | Yes, but you may have to modify your favorite positions to accommodate your pain (**»below**). Depending on the type of back pain you have, you should try placing a pillow or rolled-up towel under your pelvis for extra support and comfort. You may also find that a hot bath or gentle massage before sex can help relax your muscles and ease pain.

Q | What do I do if my partner has back pain?

A | If either one of you has back or neck problems, it is likely to affect both of you. Sex can be difficult or painful, causing frustration and distress to both parties. Try to open up the channels of communication so that you can discuss how you feel. Reassure your partner and make it clear that you want to work together to find a way to restore a fulfilling sex life that gives both of you pleasure.

Q | How can I tell my partner I'm in pain?

A | Back pain can be stressful as well as debilitating. Because back pain is invisible, it can be hard for your partner to fully understand your pain. Talking to your partner about your discomfort is very important: describe your pain as clearly as possible and explain that you are still attracted to him or her but that the pain in your back is causing you distress.

Q | How can we make sure sex is still special?

A | Set aside some time when you know that neither of you will be interrupted and find a comfortable environment. Be gentle and tune into each other's feelings and reactions: honesty, support, and reassurance will go a long way to restoring your sexual relationship. Explore other forms of sensuality as part of your sex life, and spend more time on kissing and stroking. There are many ways to enjoy a fulfilling physical relationship, so it is up to you and your partner to use your creativity and imagination and explore other avenues to find activities that will not put undue stress on areas of pain.

Q | What are the least painful positions for intercourse?

A | One of the most gentle positions is known as "spoons." For this, the female partner lies on her side with the male partner directly behind her in the same position, so that their bodies fit together like spoons. The "doggie" position can work well for women who have back pain. For this, she kneels on all fours with her partner positioned behind her. For men who find it painful to straighten their backs, the seated position works well, in which he sits on a chair or the edge of the bed with his partner straddling him, face to face.

TURNING IN BED

If you need to turn in bed from one side to the other, start by turning your upper arm and head—this is the natural way that babies and toddlers turn over. Your arm will initiate the movement of your upper trunk.

As you begin to roll onto your back, move your other arm in the same direction. Your pelvis will follow the movements of your arms and trunk without putting any strain on your back.

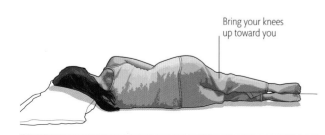

Bring your knees
up toward you

1 If you are lying on your side and want to roll over onto your back or your other side, start by bringing your knees up toward you until they are at right angles.

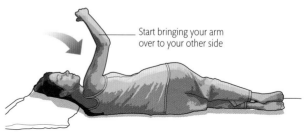

Start bringing your arm
over to your other side

2 To roll over onto your back, bring your top arm over while turning your head at the same time.

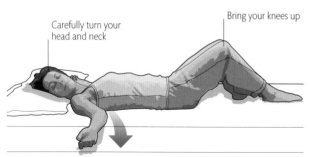

Carefully turn your
head and neck

Bring your knees up

3 Bring your legs over so that your feet and back are flat on the mattress. Your leading arm should lie out to the side you are turning toward.

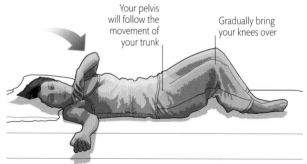

Your pelvis
will follow the
movement of
your trunk

Gradually bring
your knees over

4 Now bring your other arm over and drop your legs toward the mattress. As you do this, your head and torso will turn too.

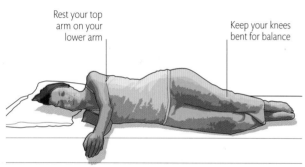

Rest your top
arm on your
lower arm

Keep your knees
bent for balance

5 Bring your arm over until it rests on your other arm, and rest your legs on the mattress. Practice this during the day so that it becomes your habit during the nighttime.

SLEEPING PROBLEMS

You may find that back pain interrupts your sleeping patterns and leads to insomnia. Follow these steps to readjust your sleeping habits:

■ Lie down to sleep only when you feel sleepy.
■ Do not do anything in bed (apart from sexual activity) except sleep.
■ If you do not fall asleep within 15 minutes of getting into bed, get up and leave the room. Do not return to bed until you are sleepy.
■ Set the alarm for the same time every morning. When it goes off, get up, regardless of how much sleep you've had.
■ Avoid naps during the day.
■ Cut down on tea, coffee, and other stimulants.
■ If you and your partner prefer different types of mattress, buy two separate mattresses and place them next to each other.

GETTING IN AND OUT OF BED

To get into bed, sit on the bed with your arms on either side of you. Lower yourself down onto one side by leaning on your elbow and then putting your head down onto the pillow, while at the same time raising your legs up onto the bed. To get out of bed, try the sequence in reverse: lie on your side and raise your head from the pillow, put your legs down onto the floor and use your arm to lift yourself up into a sitting position.

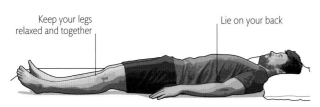

Keep your legs relaxed and together

Lie on your back

1 If you usually sleep on your front or side, turn over so that you are lying on your back, with your arms resting on either side of your body and your legs together.

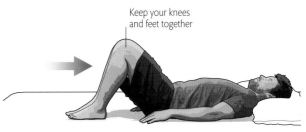

Keep your knees and feet together

2 Bring your feet toward you so that your knees are at right angles.

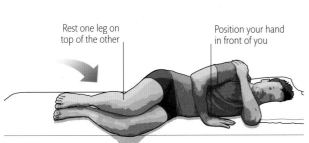

Rest one leg on top of the other

Position your hand in front of you

3 Lower your bended knees toward the edge of the bed. Rest the hand of your top arm in front of you and position your other arm so that your elbow is on the mattress and your hand is resting on your top shoulder.

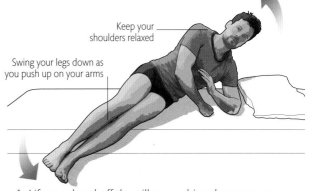

Keep your shoulders relaxed

Swing your legs down as you push up on your arms

4 Lift your head off the pillow, pushing down on your elbow and supporting hand at the same time, while bringing your feet over the edge of the bed.

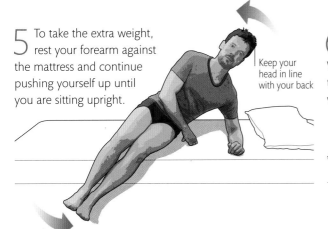

5 To take the extra weight, rest your forearm against the mattress and continue pushing yourself up until you are sitting upright.

Keep your head in line with your back

6 Place your arms either side of your body. With your feet firmly on the floor, stand up as you would from a chair.

Shift your body to the edge of the bed before you try to get up

WASHING AND DRESSING

You can make washing and dressing easier by incorporating simple coping strategies into your daily routine. For instance, when you are standing at the sink to wash, shave, or brush your teeth, avoid bending or leaning over it; as always, it is best to try to stand up straight.

If you have to stand at the sink for any length of time, try putting one hand on the basin to support your weight, and bend from your hips, not at your waist. Keep your head up and your back straight throughout. You might prefer to wash your face with a washcloth.

USING THE SHOWER AND BATH
You may find it easier to stand in the shower than sit in a bath. Put a rubber nonslip mat in the shower to keep you from slipping. Keep your toiletries in a wall rack to avoid having to bend or reach for them. Use a sponge or long-handled brush to wash with; the latter is particularly useful for washing hard-to-reach areas, such as your back and feet. If you would rather have a bath, avoid lying with your back in a rounded position for too long, because getting out may be difficult. You may find a handheld shower head useful when washing your hair. Fit a handrail to the bath if you have chronic back trouble to help you get out of the bath more easily. You may prefer to dry yourself by using a toweling dressing gown rather than a towel.

USING THE TOILET
A raised seat can make it easier for you to sit on the toilet, especially if you are tall. Lower yourself down onto the seat carefully by bending your knees and steadying yourself with a hand placed against a wall or holding onto a door in front of you. Be careful not to twist or reach around behind while you are sitting on the toilet.

YOUR MORNING ROUTINE

Washing your face and brushing your teeth are part of your daily washing routine. If you suffer from back pain, it is important you do not hunch over the sink.

Stay upright, and, if you do need to bend, bend from your hips and knees. Your toiletries should be within easy reach to avoid unnecessary reaching or bending.

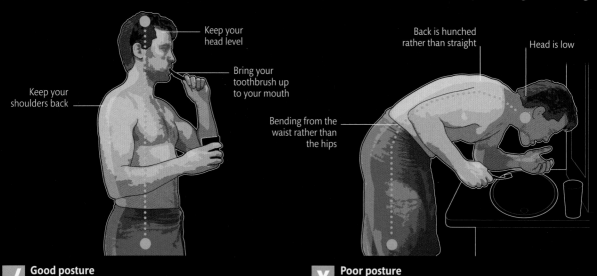

Keep your head level

Bring your toothbrush up to your mouth

Keep your shoulders back

Back is hunched rather than straight

Head is low

Bending from the waist rather than the hips

✓ Good posture
When brushing your teeth at the sink, stand upright rather than crouched over the sink. You may find it easier to use a cup filled with water to rinse out your mouth. If you shave, the mirror should be directly in front of you. An extendable mirror to the side of the basin may also be handy

✗ Poor posture
To rinse your mouth out, do not be tempted to bend at your waist because this could aggravate a back injury. Instead, bend from your hips and bend your knees, keeping your back in a neutral position to take the stress off your spine

WASHING AND DRESSING Q&A

Q Should I shower, or bathe?

A If you are experiencing acute pain, and/or suffering from disk problems, you should shower instead of taking a bath. This will prevent you from bending your back for a prolonged period and aggravating the condition. Take care when stepping in and out of the shower—a nonslip mat will help prevent accidents.

Q How can I wash my back properly?

A It can be tricky reaching all parts of your body, your back in particular. A long-handled body brush will reach areas that would otherwise be hard to get to.

Q How do I wash my feet?

A Stand on a mat next to the shower or bath, and place one foot on the side of the tub. If you are able to bathe, bring your foot up toward you while lying in the bath.

Q What sort of clothing should I wear?

A Loose clothing that is easy to put on and take off and that does not restrict your movement is always a good option. Tops with a zipper or buttons are good for the same reasons.

Q What type of shoes should I wear?

A Shoes without laces are easy to slip on and off. Women should avoid wearing high heels because these can cause lower-back pain. If in doubt, choose comfortable footwear that requires the least possible amount of effort.

Q Can I wear boots?

A You should avoid wearing boots or any other kind of heavy or stiff footwear that requires you to apply unnecessary force to put them on or take them off (»**above**).

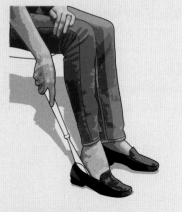

Putting on shoes
A long-handled shoe horn is a useful tool when bending over is painful. Simply sit on a chair and use the shoehorn to ease your foot into the shoe.

GETTING DRESSED

You should try to avoid having to bend your back while dressing—instead, lie flat or stand up straight. In general, it is best to avoid wearing tight clothing that restricts your movement. You will also find slip-on shoes much easier to put on and take off.

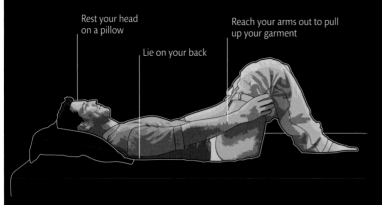

Rest your head on a pillow

Lie on your back

Reach your arms out to pull up your garment

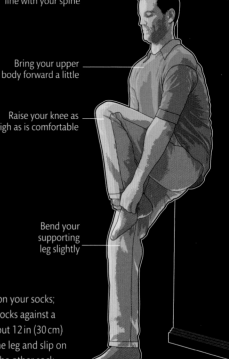

Keep your head in line with your spine

Bring your upper body forward a little

Raise your knee as high as is comfortable

Bend your supporting leg slightly

Putting on underwear and trousers
You may find putting on underwear or trousers more comfortable when performed lying down. Step into your trousers and carefully move onto the bed, taking care not to bend, and lie down on your back. Raise your hips off the bed slightly to pull your garment all the way up. To remove the garment, reverse the sequence.

Putting on socks
Don't sit down to put on your socks; instead, lean your buttocks against a wall with your feet about 12 in (30 cm) from the wall. Raise one leg and slip on your sock. Repeat for the other sock.

MOVING AROUND

When performing everyday tasks such as household chores, personal care, or social activities, it is important to maintain good neck and back posture so you can continue your daily life without putting undue stress on your back.

Additionally, it is a good idea to help yourself by making use of the many mobility aids available to simplify routine tasks, whether in the home or outside (**»opposite**).

HOME AND GARDEN

Nobody knows your home as well as you do. There may be areas that you know could be made more accessible: make a note of these and aim to make the necessary changes. For instance, you may find you have to reach beyond your comfortable range to access an everyday item in the kitchen; or you may need to crouch down to get to the cleaning products in the bathroom. As a general rule, put objects that you use more frequently at an easily accessible height so that you do not have to bend, stretch, twist, or lift unnecessarily.

In the garden, use long-handled tools, and if you need to do labor-intensive work such as digging or shoveling, take the necessary precautions (**»pp.54–55**).

If you find that you are struggling to make your home more user-friendly, an occupational therapist will be able to assess your home in relation to your needs and advise you on how best to adapt it. The therapist will also be able to teach you new ways of doing things.

SOCIAL ACTIVITIES

Some social activities may require you to stand on your feet for hours on end, leading to back pain and aching joints. Wear flat, comfortable shoes, take regular rests, and, if you are attending an event where seating will not always be available, take your own portable stool with you (**»opposite**).

GETTING OUT OF AN ARMCHAIR

It is important to learn how to get out of an armchair safely to avoid potential back injuries and falls. If you suffer from back pain, using your arms to help raise yourself up will relieve stress on your lower back.

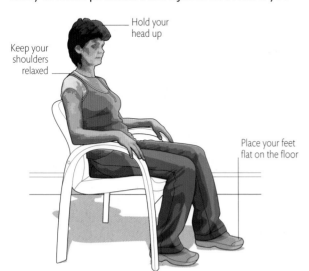

Hold your head up

Keep your shoulders relaxed

Place your feet flat on the floor

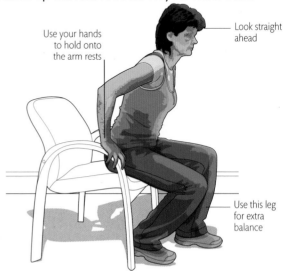

Use your hands to hold onto the arm rests

Look straight ahead

Use this leg for extra balance

1 When you are ready to stand up, place your arms and hands on the arm rests. Make sure your feet are flat on the floor about hip-distance apart, with one foot positioned slightly in front of the other for balance.

2 Move your buttocks toward the edge of the chair. Lean forward until your nose is above your knees and use your arms to help push yourself up. Keep your head, shoulders, and back aligned.

MOBILITY AIDS

A range of mobility aids can reduce the strain of everyday activities and ease chronic back pain and knee joint stress. For instance, if you struggle to reach high or low objects, a compact reaching aid will extend your reach so that you can pick up items easily without straining your back. Collapsible walking sticks are lightweight, compact, and can be stored away when not in use. Portable folding stools are ideal for when you are working in low, uncomfortable positions, such as tending the garden, where you would otherwise be on your knees, bending or crouching in awkward positions.

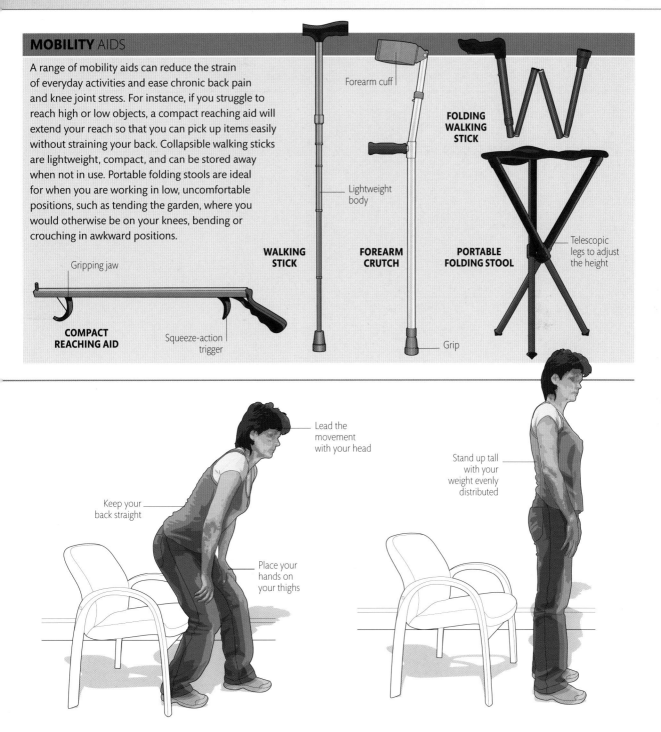

Forearm cuff

Lightweight body

FOLDING WALKING STICK

Telescopic legs to adjust the height

Gripping jaw

WALKING STICK

FOREARM CRUTCH

PORTABLE FOLDING STOOL

COMPACT REACHING AID

Squeeze-action trigger

Grip

Lead the movement with your head

Keep your back straight

Place your hands on your thighs

Stand up tall with your weight evenly distributed

3 As you push yourself up, gradually straighten your legs and let go of the arm rests. Place your hands on your thighs to support your weight and keep your head in line with your back throughout the move.

4 Continue straightening your legs until you are fully upright, and move your back leg forward so that your feet are together.

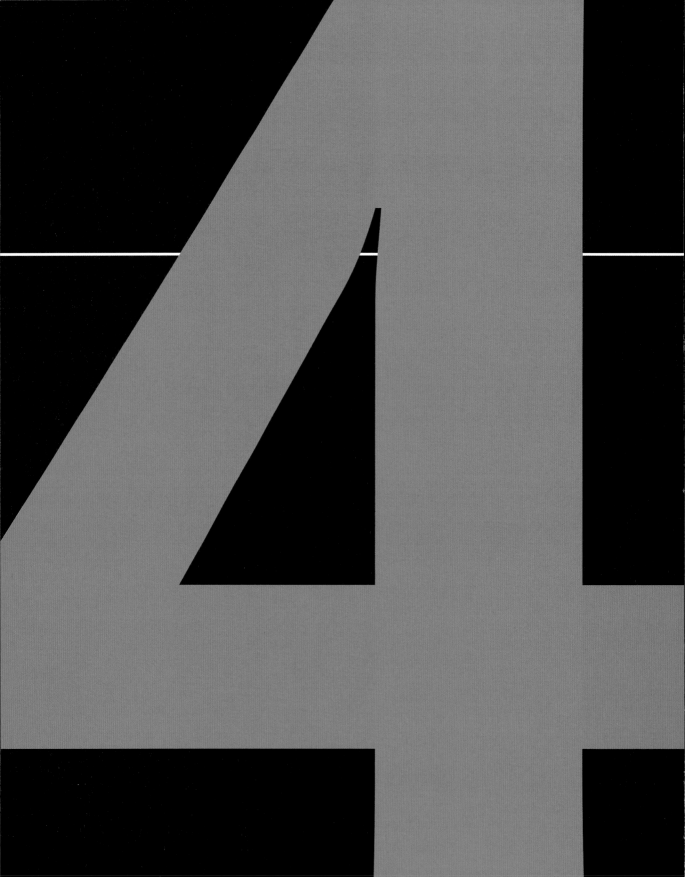

MAINTENANCE & REHABILITATION EXERCISES

This chapter guides you step by step through a wide range of exercises that your physical therapist may recommend as part of your recovery program. Most of them can also be used as part of a general fitness regimen to increase your overall flexibility, mobility, and strength, reduce your body fat, and improve your posture, all of which can help reduce your chances of back and neck trouble. Be sure to consult your doctor and physical therapist before beginning any exercise program, and follow the general safety guidelines in this book (>>p.128).

NECK AND BACK

Improving the mobility and strength in your back and neck is one of the best ways to help prevent problems occurring in the first place, because this improves your posture and reduces muscular tension. Performed as part of a rehabilitation program, exercises can help with recovery from acute conditions and may help if you have chronic pain.

1 NECK ROTATION

This simple movement helps ease neckache, maintain neck flexibility, and delay or prevent age-related stiffness. You should be able to rotate your neck through 70–90 degrees on either side without straining.

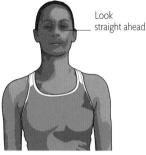
Look straight ahead

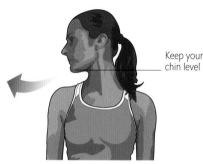
Keep your chin level

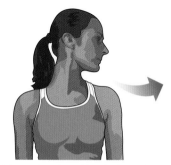

1 Look straight ahead, keeping your spine in a neutral position. Keep your upper body relaxed and your arms loose by your sides.

2 Move your head slowly to the side to look over your right shoulder. Turn it as far as is comfortable and hold for a few seconds.

3 Move your head back through the starting position, until you are looking over your left shoulder, without straining. Return to the start position.

2 NECK SIDE FLEXION

This useful mobility exercise is ideal if you suffer from aching muscles in your upper back and neck. Poor posture or an awkward sleeping position can result in imbalances in the muscles of your neck and shoulders. This may cause pain or even headaches, and is a common condition in desk workers.

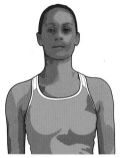

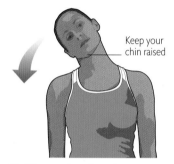
Keep your chin raised

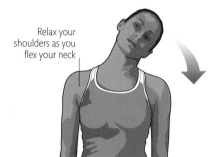
Relax your shoulders as you flex your neck

1 Stand upright, holding your body in a relaxed posture, with your shoulders loose and your eyes looking straight ahead.

2 Tilt your head so that your right ear moves toward your right shoulder as far as is comfortable. Hold for a few seconds.

3 Flex your neck in the opposite direction as far as you can go. Hold for a few seconds and return to the start position.

3 NECK EXTENSION AND FLEXION

This easy movement, which can be carried out either standing or seated, will help prevent a build-up of tension in your neck and upper-back muscles, and mobilizes the joints and nerves in your neck.

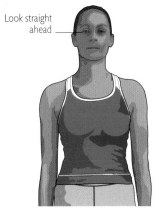
Look straight ahead

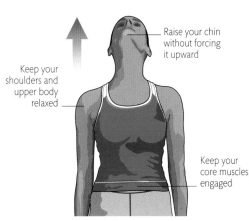
Keep your shoulders and upper body relaxed

Raise your chin without forcing it upward

Keep your core muscles engaged

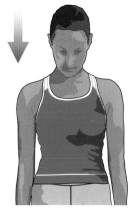

1 Stand upright with your arms by your sides in a relaxed posture. Look straight ahead and keep your spine in a neutral position.

2 Extend your neck as far as is comfortable by slowly raising your chin so you are looking directly upward. Hold for a few seconds.

3 Flex your neck by letting your head drop forward without straining. Hold for a few seconds and return to the start position.

4 SHOULDER ROTATION

If you have a stiff neck, you will benefit from this exercise, which loosens the muscles in the head, neck, and shoulder areas. It also helps to increase mobility in your neck and shoulders.

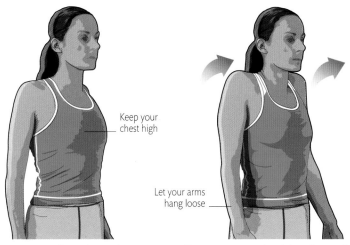
Keep your chest high

Let your arms hang loose

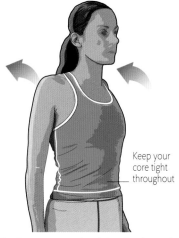
Keep your core tight throughout

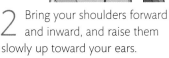

1 Let your arms hang loose by your sides and relax your shoulders. Keep your head level and your spine in a neutral position.

2 Bring your shoulders forward and inward, and raise them slowly up toward your ears.

3 Rotate your shoulders backward and around to the start position, still looking straight ahead.

5 NEURAL GLIDE

Also known as "flossing," this exercise is great for helping with neural tension in your spine and legs. When you are starting off, be gentle and don't push yourself too hard—you will develop the range of movement eventually.

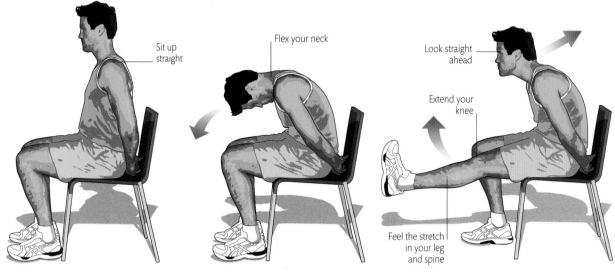

Sit up straight

Flex your neck

Look straight ahead

Extend your knee

Feel the stretch in your leg and spine

1 Sit on a chair, with your back straight, your spine lengthened, and your arms tucked behind your back, with your hands resting on the chair.

2 Slump forward and down, so that your spine is rounded and your neck is flexed.

3 Straighten your left leg as far as is comfortable and, at the same time, lift your head. Hold the position for 5 seconds. Return to the position in Step 2 and repeat with your right leg.

6 UPPER-BACK STRETCH

This easy stretch specifically mobilizes the muscles in your upper back, making it a useful rehabilitation movement for those recovering from injuries to that area, as well as a good warm-up for any activity involving your shoulders.

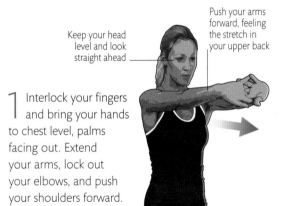

Keep your head level and look straight ahead

Push your arms forward, feeling the stretch in your upper back

1 Interlock your fingers and bring your hands to chest level, palms facing out. Extend your arms, lock out your elbows, and push your shoulders forward. Hold for 30 seconds.

7 PEC STRETCH

This stretch targets the pectoral muscles of your upper chest, easing any tightness to help increase flexibility and movement in your shoulders and upper back.

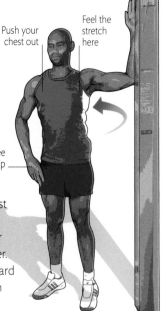

Push your chest out

Feel the stretch here

Rest your free hand on your hip

1 Stand sideways close to a solid vertical support. Rest one arm behind the upright support, keeping your upper arm in line with your shoulder. Rock your body gently forward until you can feel the stretch in your chest.

8 **MANUAL** ISOMETRICS

These neck-strengthening exercises use your hands for resistance and can be performed either standing or sitting down. These are essential exercises if you have suffered a neck injury or are starting to strengthen your neck. As you progress, you can use bands or a pulley machine to provide the required resistance.

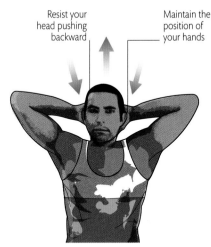

Resist your head pushing backward

Maintain the position of your hands

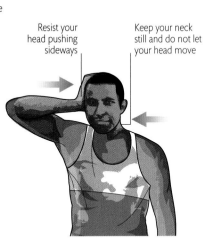

Resist your head pushing sideways

Keep your neck still and do not let your head move

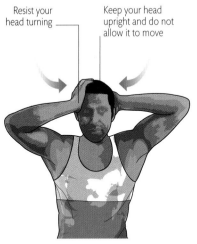

Resist your head turning

Keep your head upright and do not allow it to move

1 Clasp your hands behind your head. Press your head backward against them, resisting with your hands and ensuring that your head doesn't move. Hold for 6 seconds, then relax.

2 Hold the heel of your hand against the side of your head and press your head sideways against it, while resisting with your arm. Hold for 6 seconds, relax, then switch hands and direction.

3 Press your right hand to your temple and your left hand to the back of your head. Turn your head to the right, resisting with both arms. Hold for 6 seconds, relax, then switch hands and direction.

9 **TRUNK** ROTATION

Rotating the trunk of your body to each side will gently work the muscles around your spine. You should be able to feel the stretch in your upper back as you turn in either direction, but do not push the movement too hard.

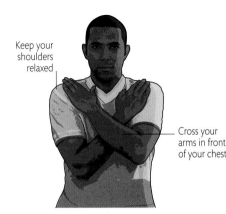

Keep your shoulders relaxed

Cross your arms in front of your chest

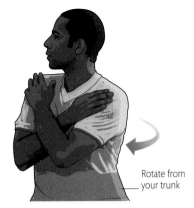

Rotate from your trunk

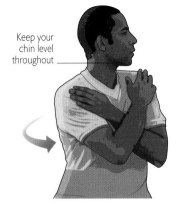

Keep your chin level throughout

1 Sit astride a chair, straighten your spine, cross your arms in front of your chest, and inhale deeply.

2 Slowly turn to your right as far as you can, exhaling as you do so, and holding the position briefly.

3 Rotate back the other way, as far as you can. Hold briefly and return to the start position.

10 LYING TRUNK ROTATION

This exercise helps improve the rotational mobility of your upper-back muscles and your thoracic spine, while stretching the muscles of your chest.

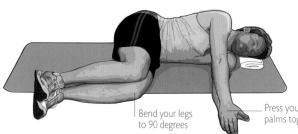

Bend your legs to 90 degrees

Press your palms together

1 Lie on your left side with your hips, knees, and feet stacked one above the other, and your hips and knees bent at right angles. Extend your arms straight in front of you, pressing your palms together.

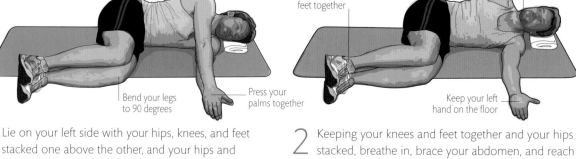

Keep your right arm straight as you reach upward

Rotate your head at the same time

Keep your feet together

Keep your left hand on the floor

2 Keeping your knees and feet together and your hips stacked, breathe in, brace your abdomen, and reach upward and back with your right hand, while keeping your left arm straight and resting on the floor.

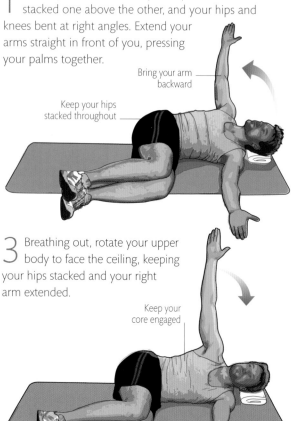

Bring your arm backward

Keep your hips stacked throughout

3 Breathing out, rotate your upper body to face the ceiling, keeping your hips stacked and your right arm extended.

Rotate your torso

4 Continue the movement until your right arm is as far back as possible, your upper body is facing up, and your hips are still stacked. Hold the movement briefly, keeping your shoulders stable and level. Breathe in.

Keep your core engaged

5 Breathing out, reach back toward the ceiling with your right arm, while rotating your torso back toward the start position slowly and under control.

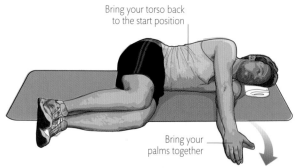

Bring your torso back to the start position

Bring your palms together

6 Continue the movement toward the start position and touch the palms of your hands together. Repeat the movement as required, then switch sides.

11 CAT STRETCH

This dynamic exercise works really well as a lower-back stretch that also works your upper back and shoulders.

It promotes spinal flexibility and increases abdominal strength. Move slowly, breathing deeply as you perform it.

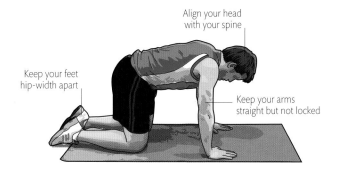

Align your head with your spine

Keep your feet hip-width apart

Keep your arms straight but not locked

1 Kneel on all fours, with your hands in line with your shoulders, your fingers pointing forward, and your knees below your hips. Keep your feet hip-width apart.

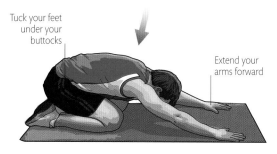

Tuck your feet under your buttocks

Extend your arms forward

2 Sit back onto your heels and stretch your arms out in front of you, keeping your palms flat on the floor.

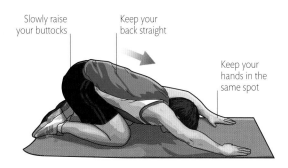

Slowly raise your buttocks

Keep your back straight

Keep your hands in the same spot

3 Slowly start to raise your buttocks, sliding your body forward while lowering your forehead toward the mat. Keep your hands in position and flat on the floor.

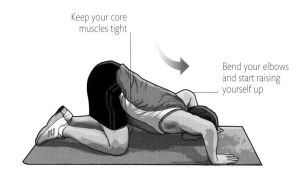

Keep your core muscles tight

Bend your elbows and start raising yourself up

4 As you continue to raise your buttocks, bend your elbows and start raising your upper body.

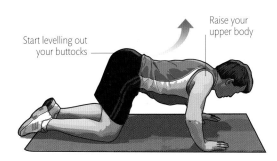

Start levelling out your buttocks

Raise your upper body

5 Continue lifting yourself up, gradually straightening your elbows and back. Keep your head level with your back.

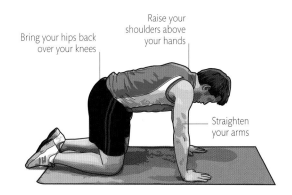

Bring your hips back over your knees

Raise your shoulders above your hands

Straighten your arms

6 Continue the movement until you return to the start position. Repeat the exercise for the required number of reps.

12 **SHOULDER** SHRUG

If you have a stiff and painful neck, this exercise is helpful for releasing tension in those muscles closest to your head.

Raise your shoulders as high as you can: you will really feel the stretch in your neck when you lower them.

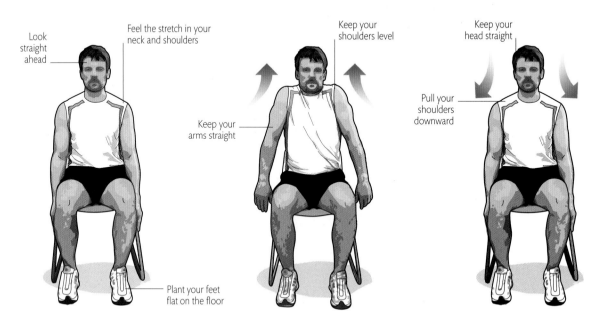

Look straight ahead

Feel the stretch in your neck and shoulders

Keep your arms straight

Plant your feet flat on the floor

Keep your shoulders level

Keep your head straight

Pull your shoulders downward

1 Sit on a chair with your knees at right angles and your feet hip-width apart. Let your shoulders drop, and your arms hang by your sides.

2 Raise your shoulders upward as high as you can, keeping your elbows as straight as possible.

3 Hold the position for around 5 seconds, then relax to return to the start position. Repeat for the required number of reps.

13 **PRONE BREAST** STROKE

This exercise strengthens the muscles of your upper back and is recommended for scoliosis, hypermobility, and relieving postural upper-back pain.

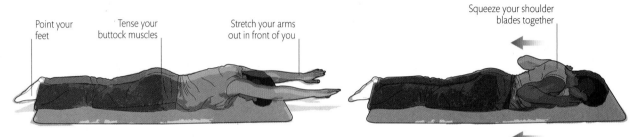

Point your feet

Tense your buttock muscles

Stretch your arms out in front of you

Squeeze your shoulder blades together

1 Lie face-down on a mat with your feet touching and your buttocks contracted. Hold your neck in a neutral position off the mat and stretch your arms forward past your head, keeping them raised off the floor and parallel. Take a deep breath in.

2 With your arms still raised, bring them back close to your chest, slowly and under control, bending your elbows and keeping them at the same level as your hands, squeezing your shoulder blades together. Breathe out. Repeat for the required number of reps, then relax.

14 PRONE SHOULDER SQUEEZE

This exercise strengthens your upper back and the back of your shoulders, and helps to improve your posture. It is a useful movement for people with rounded back and shoulders, which is common in desk workers.

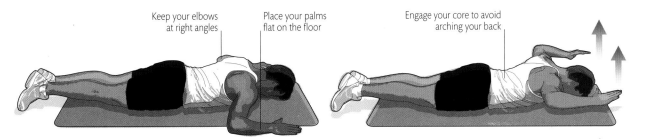

Keep your elbows at right angles

Place your palms flat on the floor

Engage your core to avoid arching your back

1 Lie face-down with your forehead resting on a mat and your elbows at right angles, palms facing down and on the floor. Point your feet back, with your toes on the floor.

2 Raise your arms off the floor to head height and squeeze your shoulder blades together. Return to the start position and repeat for the required number of reps.

15 SEATED SHOULDER SQUEEZE

This exercise mobilizes the muscles and nerves of your upper back and shoulders, and is ideal for people in sedentary or desk-based jobs. It can also help prevent repetitive strain injury (RSI), and can ease cases of pain in your hands and forearms. Aim to perform 10 reps 5 or 6 times per day.

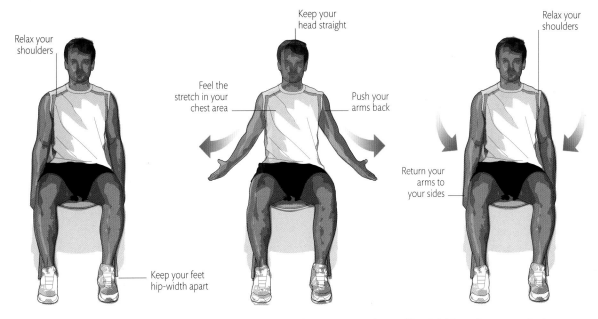

Relax your shoulders

Keep your head straight

Relax your shoulders

Feel the stretch in your chest area

Push your arms back

Return your arms to your sides

Keep your feet hip-width apart

1 Sit on a backless seat with your back straight, your arms hanging loosely by your sides, and your feet hip-width apart and flat on the floor.

2 With your palms facing out, push your arms backward and away from your body as far as you can go without straining.

3 Hold for a few seconds then return to the start position, slowly and under control. Repeat for the required number of reps.

16 LEVATOR SCAPULAE STRETCH

This simple stretch involves using the weight of your head to stretch your neck muscles. It offers instant relief from tense neck and shoulder muscles and can be a useful exercise for desk workers.

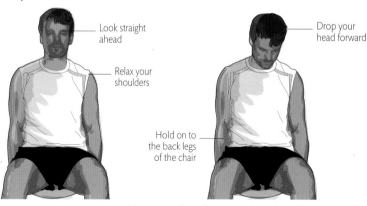

Look straight ahead

Relax your shoulders

Hold on to the back legs of the chair

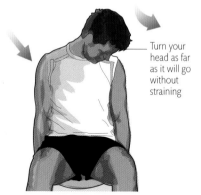

Drop your head forward

Turn your head as far as it will go without straining

1 Sit unsupported on a chair with your shoulders aligned and your arms straight. Grip the underside or the back legs of the chair with your hands.

2 Allow your head to drop down as far as it can without bending your upper back, then slowly turn your head toward your left shoulder.

3 Hold the position for around 5 seconds, until you feel the stretch in the muscles to the right of your neck. Return to the start position and swap sides.

17 DOORWAY CHEST STRETCH

Similar to the corner chest stretch (»p.84), this exercise mobilizes the muscles and nerves in your arms and improves mobility in your shoulder blades. Perform this movement slowly and fluidly.

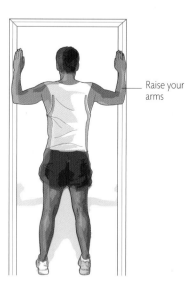

Keep your head in line with your spine

Press your palms against the doorframe

Raise your arms

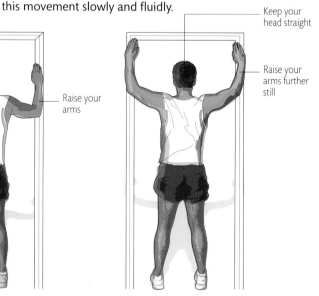

Keep your head straight

Raise your arms further still

1 Stand in a doorway, with your feet hip-width apart, and your hands at shoulder height and resting flat against the doorframe.

2 Slowly and with control, slide your hands up the doorframe, until your elbows are bent at right angles.

3 Continue the movement until your elbows are at shoulder height. Reverse the movement to return to the start position.

18 SUPINE NECK FLEXION

This is a mobilizing exercise, which activates the deep muscles of your neck along with the upper and lower joints of your neck. It is often used in the rehabilitation of whiplash injuries and tension headaches.

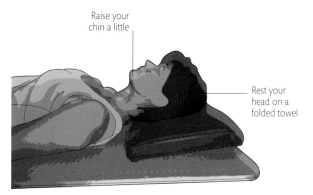

Raise your chin a little

Rest your head on a folded towel

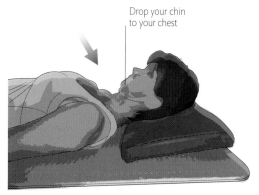

Drop your chin to your chest

1 Lie on your back with your head supported by a folded towel, your pelvis and upper back relaxed, and your arms resting either side of your body. Lift your chin a little so that your face points slightly upward.

2 Slowly slide the back of your head up the towel until the plane of your face tilts forward as far as it will go and your chin drops all the way toward your throat. Hold for a few seconds then return to the start position.

19 NECK EXTENSION WITH OVERPRESSURE

This is a mobilizing exercise for your neck that is used in the rehabilitation of most neck conditions. You should perform it in one fluid movement for no more than 10 reps 5 or 6 times per day. If you experience pain or pins and needles in your arm while doing the exercise, you should stop immediately and consult your therapist.

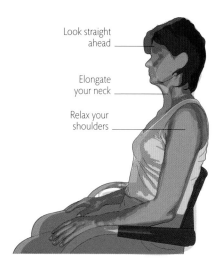
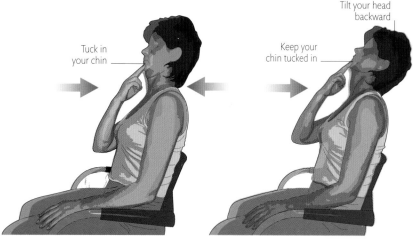

Look straight ahead

Elongate your neck

Relax your shoulders

Tuck in your chin

Tilt your head backward

Keep your chin tucked in

1 Sit in a chair and rest your arms on your thighs. Keeping your head straight, drop your shoulders and elongate your neck.

2 Applying gentle pressure with your hand, tuck your chin in. Your neck and head will shift backwards automatically.

3 Keeping your chin tucked in, extend your neck by bending it backward in one fluid movement. Hold this position for no more than 2 seconds, then return to the start position.

20 **UPPER-BACK** EXTENSION

This stretching movement works the muscles of your upper back and shoulders. It helps support your spine and improve your posture, and is a good exercise for desk workers.

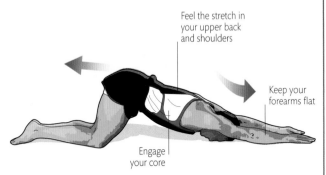

Feel the stretch in your upper back and shoulders

Keep your forearms flat

Engage your core

1 Kneel on an exercise mat and lower your body forward slowly and carefully, extending your arms forward so that your forehead touches the mat. Press down against the floor with your hands and forearms, and ease your buttocks backward as far as you can. Pause at the edge of the movement, then relax to return to the start position.

21 **SWISS BALL** BACK STRETCH

This exercise stretches the joints of your upper and lower back, and helps to improve the alignment of your spinal joints.

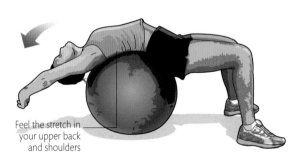

Feel the stretch in your upper back and shoulders

1 With your feet shoulder-width apart and flat on the floor, squat down onto a Swiss ball, and lean back over it so that both your shoulders and buttocks are resting on it. Stretch both arms over your head and allow your arms to fall as far as they will go. Hold the position for a few seconds, breathing in and out, then return to the start position.

22 **SEATED BACK** EXTENSION

This stretch helps to loosen tight muscles in your upper back, while working those that support your spine, improving your posture and helping to ease the muscle tension that can result from working at a desk or long periods of sitting. The exercise can be performed in most chairs, making it a versatile and easy movement, and is especially recommended to those in sedentary jobs, or who suffer from a stiff neck and upper back.

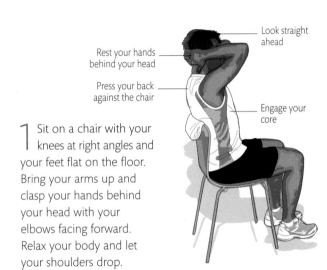

Look straight ahead

Rest your hands behind your head

Press your back against the chair

Engage your core

Keep your elbows in line

Push your chest out

1 Sit on a chair with your knees at right angles and your feet flat on the floor. Bring your arms up and clasp your hands behind your head with your elbows facing forward. Relax your body and let your shoulders drop.

2 Extend your elbows backward, keeping them at shoulder height. Breathe in and push your chest forward and upward while arching your spine. Pause, then return to the start position.

23 UPPER-BACK BAND ROW

This exercise works the muscles of your shoulders and upper back, and is recommended to those who suffer from postural strain or scoliosis. Loop the resistance band safely through a door handle or similar.

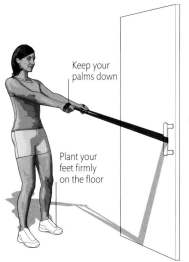

Keep your palms down

Plant your feet firmly on the floor

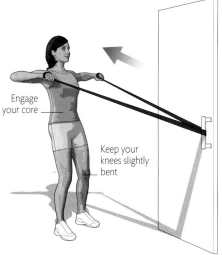

Engage your core

Keep your knees slightly bent

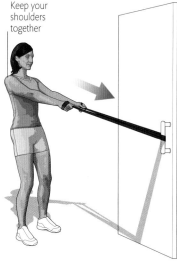

Keep your shoulders together

1 Hold the ends of the band with your arms extended. Squeeze your shoulder blades down and together, and inhale.

2 Exhale as you pull the band to shoulder height, bending your elbows out to the sides.

3 Inhale as you release the band and return to the start position. Repeat several times.

24 LAT BAND ROW

This exercise works the large muscles of your upper back and the back of your shoulders. It is particularly effective for sufferers of postural strain or scoliosis. Keep your feet in the same spot throughout.

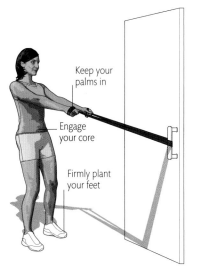

Keep your palms in

Engage your core

Firmly plant your feet

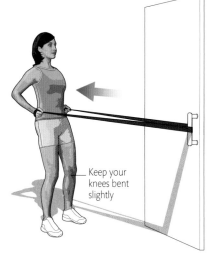

Keep your knees bent slightly

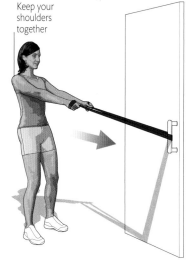

Keep your shoulders together

1 Hold the ends of the band with your arms extended. Squeeze your shoulder blades down and together, and inhale.

2 Exhale as you pull the band into the sides of your waist. Keep your elbows parallel.

3 Inhale as you release the band and return to the start position.

25 PASSIVE NECK RETRACTION

This is a mobilizing exercise for your neck and is especially helpful if you have a facet joint problem, disk problem, or nerve impingement in your neck. Start gently and perform no more than 10 reps 5 or 6 times a day. You may feel some discomfort, but you should stop immediately if the exercise becomes painful.

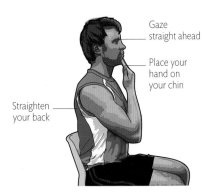

Gaze straight ahead

Place your hand on your chin

Straighten your back

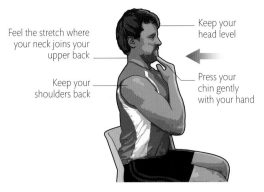

Feel the stretch where your neck joins your upper back

Keep your shoulders back

Keep your head level

Press your chin gently with your hand

1 Sit up straight with your shoulders relaxed. Look straight ahead and place your hand on your chin. Try to elongate your neck, increasing the distance between your shoulders and ears.

2 Keeping your shoulders relaxed, push your chin in with your hand, applying gentle pressure. Hold for 3 seconds, then ease the pressure and return to the start position for 3 seconds. Repeat as required.

26 ACTIVE NECK RETRACTION

Following on from the passive neck retraction exercises (»above), activating the deep muscles in your neck helps to increase the strength of the muscles responsible for good head and neck posture (»pp.36–39).

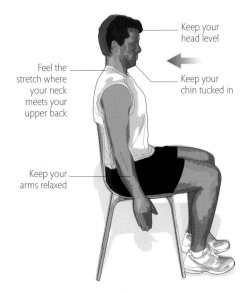

Gaze straight ahead

Relax your shoulders

Sit up straight

Keep your head level

Feel the stretch where your neck meets your upper back

Keep your chin tucked in

Keep your arms relaxed

1 Sit on a chair with your back straight and your shoulders and upper back relaxed. Look straight ahead, and allow your arms to rest at your sides with your palms toward you.

2 Tuck in your chin and elongate your neck, so that the top of your head moves upward. Hold for 5 seconds and then relax to the start position. Repeat as required.

27 **SUPINE BACK** ROTATION

This more gentle version of the back rotation (**»p.111**) improves general mobility and is useful for relaxing the muscles of your back and around your pelvis.

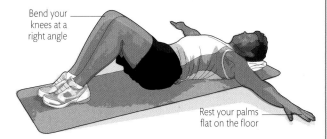

Bend your knees at a right angle

Rest your palms flat on the floor

1 Placing a folded towel under your head, if required, lie on your back with your knees together and your legs bent, your feet flat on the floor, and your arms extended with your palms facing downward.

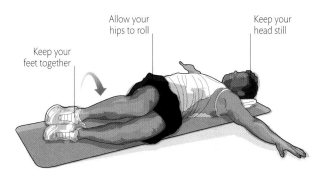

Allow your hips to roll

Keep your head still

Keep your feet together

2 Keeping your knees together, slowly roll them to your left and hold for a few seconds. Keep your upper body flat against the floor, bracing yourself with your arms.

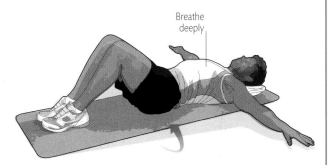

Breathe deeply

3 Slowly return to the start position. Repeat for the required number of reps before switching sides.

28 **TOWEL** ROCK

This can help a stiff or aching neck. If one side of your neck is tight, begin by rocking away from that side, then if it's not too painful, back toward the stiff side. Moving your head both ways can help restore a full range of motion.

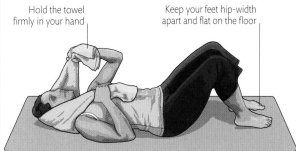

Hold the towel firmly in your hand

Keep your feet hip-width apart and flat on the floor

1 Fold a towel in three lengthwise and place it behind your head. Lie on a mat with your knees bent and your lower back pressed into the mat. If the left side of your neck is stiff, hold the left end of the towel above your head with your left hand, and the right end by your chest with your right hand.

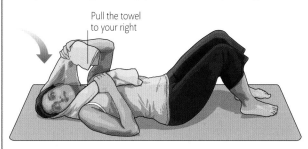

Pull the towel to your right

2 Grasping the right end firmly by your chest with your right hand, pull the left end with your left hand so that your head rocks gently to the right. Perform about 10 small rocking motions, and keep your neck muscles relaxed.

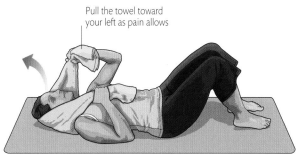

Pull the towel toward your left as pain allows

3 Return to the start position, and repeat the movements in the opposite direction if it is comfortable to do so, but don't force the movement if you feel any pain.

29 TOWEL NECK FLEXION

This self-mobilizing technique is ideal if you suffer from a stiff, painful neck, because it improves neck flexion. Let your arms do the work—your neck muscles should be fully relaxed, and the movements controlled and slow.

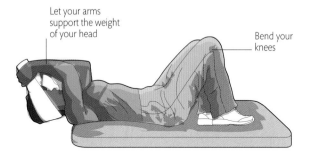

Let your arms support the weight of your head

Bend your knees

1 Lie on your back with your shoulders off the edge of a thick exercise mat or mattress. Fold a towel lengthways and place it behind your head, gripping either end to support your head and neck, which should be roughly level with your upper back. Inhale deeply.

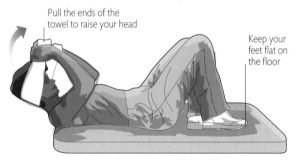

Pull the ends of the towel to raise your head

Keep your feet flat on the floor

2 Gently pull the towel forward and up. Carry the weight of your head with your arms so that your neck flexes without you using your neck muscles. Hold for 3–5 seconds and breathe out through your mouth.

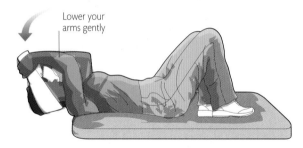

Lower your arms gently

3 Still gripping the towel, lower your arms to return to the start position slowly and under control.

30 TOWEL NECK EXTENSION

This neck exercise improves neck extension and can be done alongside the towel neck flexion exercise (»left). Remember to relax the muscles in your neck and to keep the movements slow and controlled.

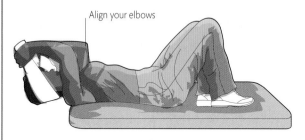

Align your elbows

1 Lie on your back with your shoulders off the edge of a thick exercise mat or mattress. Fold a towel lengthways and place it behind your head. Tightly hold the ends of the towel to support your head and neck, which should be level with your upper back. Inhale deeply.

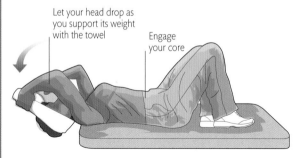

Let your head drop as you support its weight with the towel

Engage your core

2 Gripping the towel, move your arms back and down, allowing your head to drop gently. Take the weight of your head in your arms, rather than using your neck muscles. Hold for 3–5 seconds and exhale through your mouth.

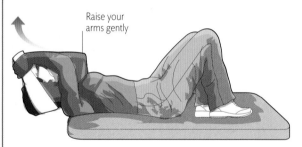

Raise your arms gently

3 Maintaining a firm grip on the towel, raise your arms slowly and under control to return to the start position.

31 OVAL SHOULDER STRETCH

This versatile exercise mobilizes your shoulders and upper back, which will improve the function of your shoulder girdle, which in turn will increase the range of motion in your upper back and prevent injuries to this area. To do this exercise correctly, perform the movement in a slow, controlled manner, and bend from your hips, not at your waist. You may also want to bend your knees slightly to take the strain from your lower back.

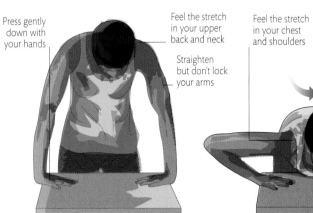

Press gently down with your hands

Feel the stretch in your upper back and neck

Straighten but don't lock your arms

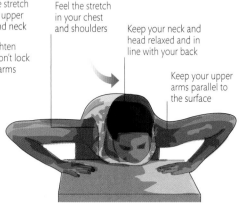

Feel the stretch in your chest and shoulders

Keep your neck and head relaxed and in line with your back

Keep your upper arms parallel to the surface

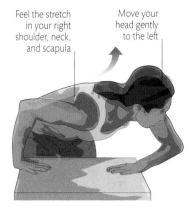

Feel the stretch in your right shoulder, neck, and scapula

Move your head gently to the left

1 Place your hands palms-down on a flat surface in front of you with your fingers slightly splayed and pointing inward. Round your upper back and tilt your head downward.

2 Keeping your hands palms-down, lower yourself until your arms are parallel to the surface and your upper body is 2 in (5 cm) above it. Slide your body left, keeping your back straight.

3 Rotate your head slowly to the left, bringing your left ear around toward your shoulder, and raise your upper body up and around toward the start position.

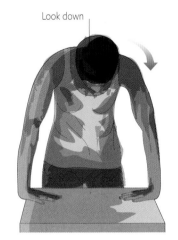

Look down

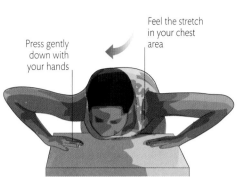

Press gently down with your hands

Feel the stretch in your chest area

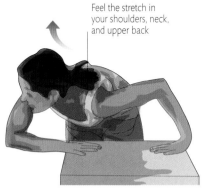

Feel the stretch in your shoulders, neck, and upper back

4 Once back in the start position, repeat the movement, but this time in the opposite direction, aiming for a slow and continuous fluid motion.

5 Lower yourself down again until your arms are parallel to the surface and your upper body is 2 in (5 cm) away from the surface. Slide your body right, keeping your back straight and your upper arms parallel to the surface.

6 Rotate your head slowly to the right and up, bringing your right ear around toward your shoulder, while lifting your upper body back to the start position. Repeat for the required number of reps in either direction, then relax.

32 ROLL-DOWN STRETCH

This exercise is an excellent stretch for your neck, but it is important to keep your head back and your chin tucked in as you roll your head down. This ensures that you stretch your entire neck, not just the lower part of it, and your upper back. It is recommended if you suffer from postural pain and tension headaches.

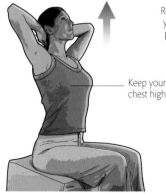
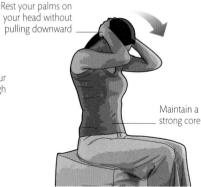

Support your head with your hands

Keep your chest high

Rest your palms on your head without pulling downward

Maintain a strong core

1 Sit slightly forward on a chair, your feet flat on the floor. Clasp your hands behind your head and press your head back into them.

2 Gently lift your gaze and look diagonally upward. Pull your elbows up and out as you stretch up, lifting your chest.

3 Tuck your chin into your neck and roll your head downward to look at your chest. Hold briefly, then roll back up to the start position.

33 CORNER CHEST STRETCH

This exercise is ideal for improving your posture, especially if the muscles of your chest and shoulders are feeling tight. To perform the stretch correctly and safely, make sure your feet are well grounded so that you can push yourself away from the wall.

VARIATION

You can vary this exercise by raising or lowering the position of your arms. By doing this you alter the stretch to focus on different parts of your chest.

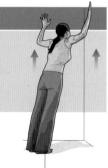

Keep your feet firmly grounded

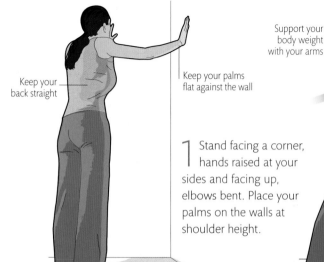

Keep your back straight

Keep your palms flat against the wall

Support your body weight with your arms

Avoid arching your back

Keep your feet flat

1 Stand facing a corner, hands raised at your sides and facing up, elbows bent. Place your palms on the walls at shoulder height.

2 Lean forward and feel the stretch in your chest and upper back between your shoulder blades. Hold this position for 15 seconds, then relax. Repeat 3 times.

34 SEATED TWIST STRETCH

This is a good exercise for the muscles around your spine. It is important to push with one arm to leverage the twist and really stretch the spine. Protect your spine by pulling your abdomen in deeply as you try to maintain the longest vertical height. Only go as far as is comfortable.

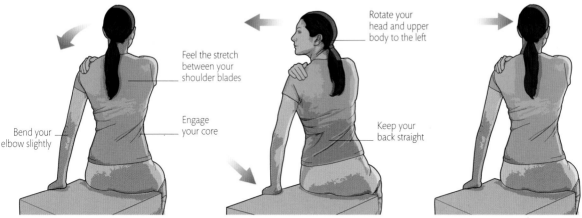

Feel the stretch between your shoulder blades

Bend your elbow slightly

Engage your core

Rotate your head and upper body to the left

Keep your back straight

1 Sit on the edge of a box or chair, your feet flat on the floor. Hold the edge of the box with your left hand, and place your right hand on your left shoulder.

2 Twist to the left, pulling your left shoulder back and pushing against the edge of the box with your left hand. Pause at the edge of the movement.

3 Relax to return to the start position. Repeat for the required number of repetitions, then swap sides.

35 SEATED WAIST STRETCH

This is a great stretch for the muscles of your upper back. To get the full benefit of the movement, elongate both sides of your torso as you reach up. Look straight ahead and try to hold yourself back in order to avoid leaning forward.

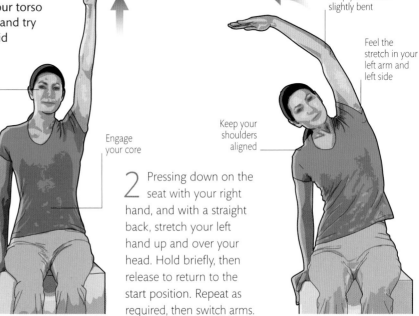

Look straight ahead of you

Engage your core

Keep your elbow slightly bent

Feel the stretch in your left arm and left side

Keep your shoulders aligned

1 Sit slightly forward on a box or chair, with your feet flat on the floor. Reach up with your left hand, palm facing inward, holding onto the edge of the box with your right hand.

2 Pressing down on the seat with your right hand, and with a straight back, stretch your left hand up and over your head. Hold briefly, then release to return to the start position. Repeat as required, then switch arms.

BACK AND BUTTOCKS

Weakness or tension in the muscles of your thighs, buttocks, and hips can cause lower-back pain, so it is important to keep them strong and mobile. Likewise, strengthening the muscles of your core improves your posture, reducing your chance of back problems. Such exercises are useful in both maintenance and the process of recovery.

36 SEATED HIP TILT

This exercise works your whole spine, from neck to pelvis, gently mobilizing your joints, muscles, and nerves. It is a good exercise for easing postural pain.

1 Sit toward the front of your seat so that your thighs slope downward a little. Rest your hands on the seat on either side of your body, with your head level. Keep your feet slightly apart and flat on the floor.

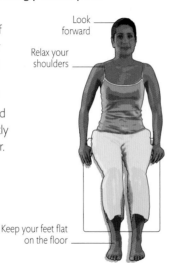

Look forward

Relax your shoulders

Keep your feet flat on the floor

2 Tilt your head to the right, while leaning your body to the left, taking the weight off your right hip bone. Hold briefly, then return to the start position. Repeat with your right side if required, this time leaning to the right and tilting your head to the left.

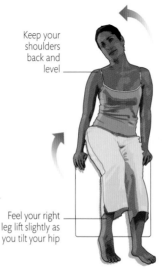

Keep your shoulders back and level

Feel your right leg lift slightly as you tilt your hip

37 SEATED HIP WALK

As with the seated hip tilt (»left), this exercise works your entire spine in multiple directions and is recommended for alleviating postural pain.

1 Sit toward the front of the seat with your thighs sloping slightly downward. Make sure you are sitting up straight with your feet flat on the floor. Line up your knees and look straight ahead.

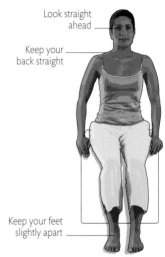

Look straight ahead

Keep your back straight

Keep your feet slightly apart

2 Press your right hip back into the seat and turn your head to the left. Hold briefly, then return to the start position. Switch sides, and repeat the movement, pressing your left hip back and turning your head to the right.

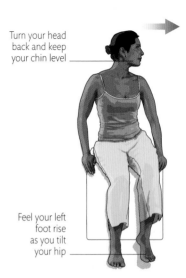

Turn your head back and keep your chin level

Feel your left foot rise as you tilt your hip

38 SQUAT

This is a key mobilizing movement for your lower body and core, and can help to improve flexibility and strength in your hips, reducing the chances of back problems occurring. Good form is crucial: go as low as possible to improve your range of motion and do not "bounce" at the bottom.

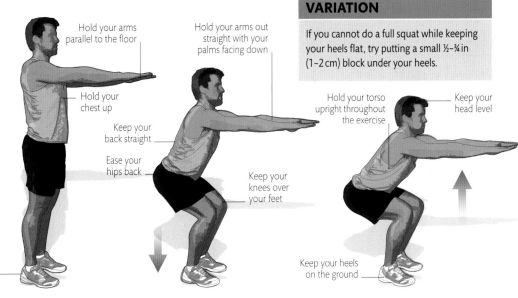

Hold your arms parallel to the floor

Hold your chest up

Hold your arms out straight with your palms facing down

Keep your back straight

Ease your hips back

Keep your knees over your feet

Place your feet shoulder-width apart

VARIATION

If you cannot do a full squat while keeping your heels flat, try putting a small ½–¾ in (1–2 cm) block under your heels.

Hold your torso upright throughout the exercise

Keep your head level

Keep your heels on the ground

1 Stand with your spine neutral, arms out in front of you, and your feet just over shoulder-width apart.

2 Inhale and, looking straight ahead, bend at your knees and hips, easing your hips backward.

3 Squat down until your thighs are parallel to the floor (or further if you can). Return to the start position.

39 WALKING LUNGE

This is an excellent way to strengthen your hips and thighs, reducing the chances of straining your back. The walking lunge tests both your balance and coordination. You can also perform it from a fixed position.

1 Stand with your feet hip-width apart and your shoulders, hips, and feet in line.

2 Take a long step forward with your right leg. Drop down and bend at your knees.

3 Push off with your left leg back to an upright position, keeping your core engaged and your head up.

4 Step forward with your left leg and drop down again. Return to the start position, repeat as required, then switch legs.

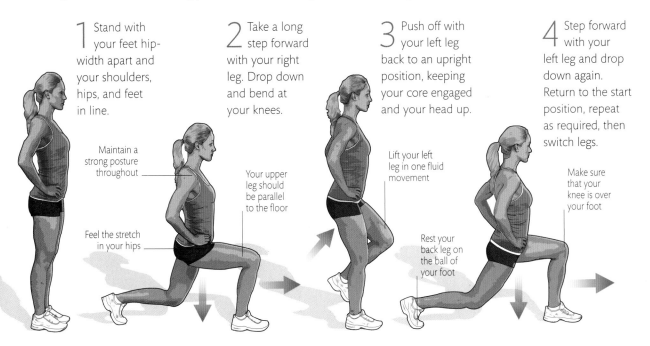

Maintain a strong posture throughout

Feel the stretch in your hips

Your upper leg should be parallel to the floor

Lift your left leg in one fluid movement

Rest your back leg on the ball of your foot

Make sure that your knee is over your foot

40 PRESS-UP

This simple exercise is a useful form of self-traction for your upper and lower back that helps elongate your spine. It can help with a range of back conditions and is a good general maintenance stretch for desk workers.

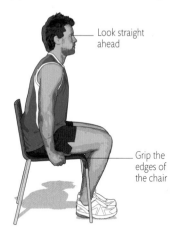

Look straight ahead

Grip the edges of the chair

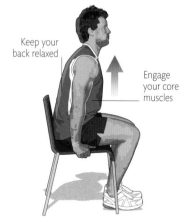

Keep your back relaxed

Engage your core muscles

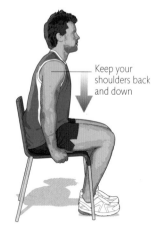

Keep your shoulders back and down

1 Sit on a chair and grip the outside edges of the seat with your hands, placing them roughly in line with your shoulders.

2 Push down with your hands and relax your back, inhaling and exhaling slowly, allowing your pelvis to drop so that your back elongates.

3 Pause briefly and lower yourself to the start position, repeating the movement as required, slowly and gently.

41 HIP-HITCHER

This exercise works the muscles around your hip joint. It is a very useful movement if you are suffering from facet joint dysfunction, and is also good for improving hip and sacroiliac joint mobility.

1 Stand upright with your left foot on a step and your right foot unsupported in the air. Place your hands on your hips for balance.

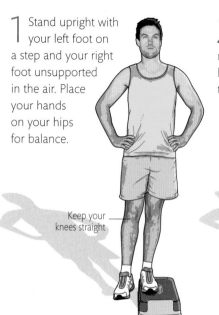

Keep your knees straight

2 Push your left hip inward, raising your right hip slightly at the same time.

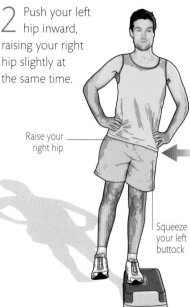

Raise your right hip

Squeeze your left buttock

3 Allow your right foot to drop down past the edge of the step, keeping your left leg as straight as you can. Pause, return to the start position, and repeat for the required number of reps before swapping sides.

Let your left hip drop outward

Lower your foot past the step

42 **WALL SIT** PRESS

This exercise is great for releasing tension in your thoracic spine, and opening up your shoulders and the muscles of your upper body.

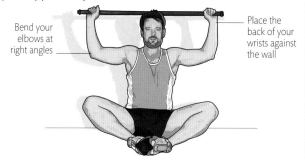

Bend your elbows at right angles

Place the back of your wrists against the wall

1 Sit with your hips, back, shoulders, elbows, wrists, and head against a wall, and the soles of your feet together. Hold a bar above your head with your elbows at 90 degrees.

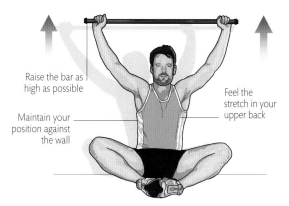

Raise the bar as high as possible

Maintain your position against the wall

Feel the stretch in your upper back

2 Slowly push the bar above your head, maintaining full contact with the wall throughout the movement.

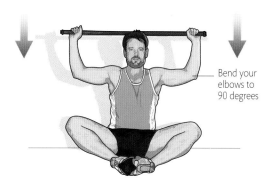

Bend your elbows to 90 degrees

3 Once you have raised the bar as far as you can, lower it back to the start position. Repeat as required.

43 CLAM

This straightforward exercise works your hip flexors and the muscles of your buttocks, while also improving overall stability in your pelvis and core.

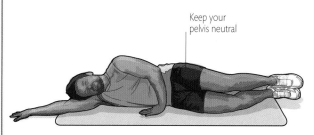

Keep your pelvis neutral

1 Lie on your right side, bending about 45 degrees at your hips and knees. Extend your right arm so that it is in line with your body, and rest your head on it. Bend your left arm at the elbow and place your left hand on the floor in front of you.

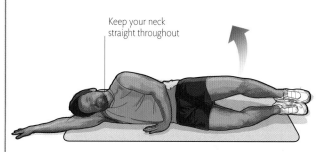

Keep your neck straight throughout

2 Keeping your neck straight, your hips and shoulders in line, and your feet touching, engage your core and begin lifting the knee of your left leg, rotating it at your hip.

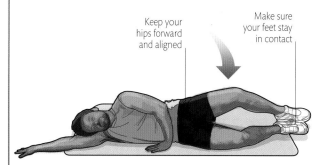

Keep your hips forward and aligned

Make sure your feet stay in contact

3 Lift your left knee as far as it will go, while keeping your hips aligned. Slowly lower your knee back to the start position, and repeat for the required number of reps before swapping sides.

44 SINGLE ARM AND LEG RAISE

This exercise engages the muscles of your core, using them to stabilize your pelvis against the motion of your arms and legs. Your core acts as a natural girdle, flattening your abdomen and supporting your lower back.

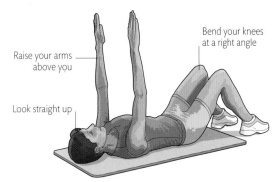

Raise your arms above you

Bend your knees at a right angle

Look straight up

1 Lie on your back with your knees bent, your feet flat on the ground, and your arms extended above you, palms facing forward. Keep your back straight and pelvis neutral.

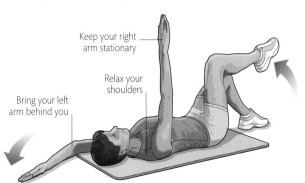

Keep your right arm stationary

Relax your shoulders

Bring your left arm behind you

2 Lower your left arm to the ground behind you as you lift your right knee above your hip, contracting your abdominals as you do so.

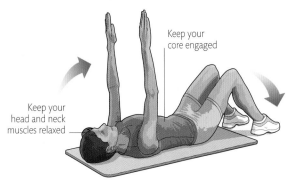

Keep your core engaged

Keep your head and neck muscles relaxed

3 Slowly return to the start position and repeat with your right arm and left leg.

45 DEAD BUG

This exercise works your lower back, pelvis, trunk, and shoulders. A moderate- to high-level Pilates exercise, it should only be attempted after mastering more basic Pilates exercises, such as the single arm and leg raise (»left). If you are recovering from a back injury, ensure that you keep your lower back pressed against the floor.

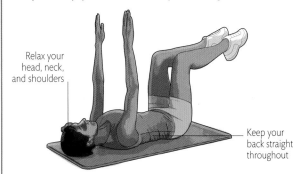

Relax your head, neck, and shoulders

Keep your back straight throughout

1 Lie on your back on a mat and contract your abdominals. Bend your hips and knees at 90 degrees, and position your feet roughly hip-width apart in the air. Point your arms up directly over your shoulders, palms facing forward.

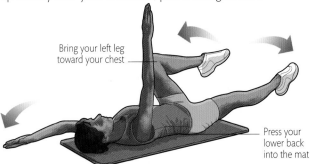

Bring your left leg toward your chest

Press your lower back into the mat

2 Lower your left arm behind you and extend your right leg, bringing it as close to the floor as possible without arching your back. Draw your left knee to your chest.

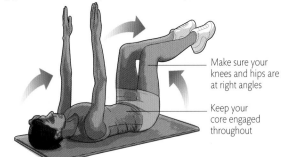

Make sure your knees and hips are at right angles

Keep your core engaged throughout

3 Briefly hold the position, ensuring you do not arch your back, then return to the start position and switch sides.

46 SACRAL CIRCLE

This exercise relaxes the muscles surrounding your sacroiliac joints, and provides a form of self-massage that helps mobilize them. It can be used to help with sacroiliac strain.

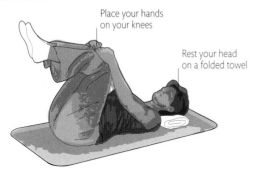

Place your hands on your knees

Rest your head on a folded towel

1 Lie on a mat, placing a folded towel under your head for support. Gently exhale as you slowly bring your knees back toward your chest and place your hands on them.

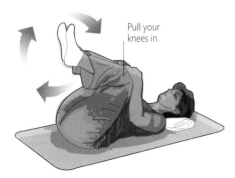

Pull your knees in

2 Circle your knees from right to left 5 times, using your hands to guide the movement. Breathe normally.

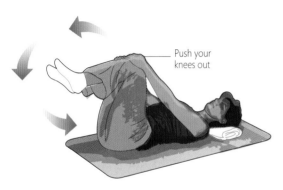

Push your knees out

3 Repeat the exercise 5 times in the opposite direction, from left to right, drawing your arms in and out as you perform the movement.

47 ONE-LEG CIRCLE

This exercise can be used as a mobilizing technique for your sciatic nerve, and can help with sciatica. The movement should be fluid and gentle.

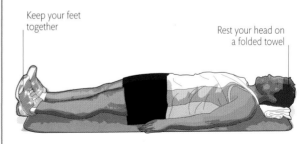

Keep your feet together

Rest your head on a folded towel

1 Lie on your back with a folded towel under your head for support. Rest your arms either side of your body.

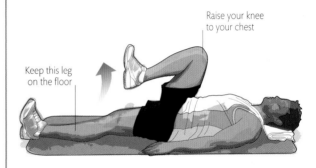

Raise your knee to your chest

Keep this leg on the floor

2 Bring your right knee to your chest, extending your foot upward toward your body as you do so.

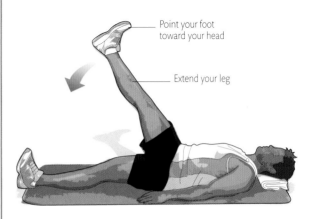

Point your foot toward your head

Extend your leg

3 Without pausing, stretch your right leg up toward the ceiling and then drop it toward the mat with control, in a circular motion. Repeat the circle for the required number of reps, then return to the start position and swap legs.

48 ALLIGATOR

This exercise mobilizes your whole spine with a side-to-side movement, and is a great exercise to increase your spinal flexibility. It should be performed in one fluid motion from one side to the other.

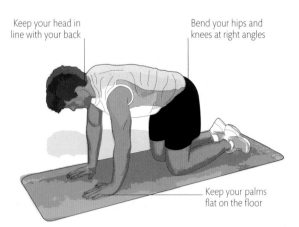

Keep your head in line with your back

Bend your hips and knees at right angles

Keep your palms flat on the floor

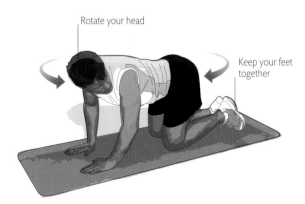

Rotate your head

Keep your feet together

1 Start on all fours with your back flat and your neck in a relaxed position. Position your arms directly under your shoulders, and bend your hips and knees at right angles. Keep your feet together. Take a deep breath in.

2 Exhaling, turn your head and pelvis to the left and toward each other, feeling the stretch along the right side of your body. Pause, then repeat the movement to your right. Complete the desired number of repetitions on either side, then relax to the start position.

49 LYING WAIST TWIST

This exercise increases the mobility of the joints and muscles in your lower and upper back. Perform the exercise 3 times on each side, holding the position for 15 seconds.

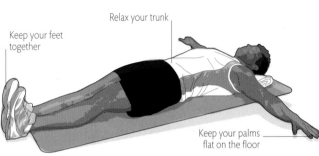

Keep your feet together

Relax your trunk

Keep your palms flat on the floor

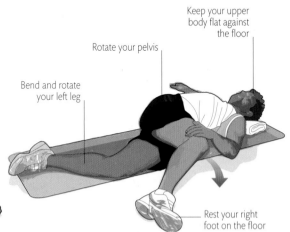

Keep your upper body flat against the floor

Rotate your pelvis

Bend and rotate your left leg

Rest your right foot on the floor

1 Placing a folded towel under your head for extra support, lie on your back, with your body relaxed and your arms loose but extended at a 90-degree angle from your upper body. Keep your legs and feet together.

2 Keeping your upper body flat against the mat, bend your right leg at the knee and bring it across your body, using your left hand to increase the stretch, and allowing your left leg to turn and bend in the same direction. Hold the move, then return to the start position and switch sides.

50 GLUTEAL/PIRIFORMIS FOAM ROLLER

This exercise loosens up the gluteals at the outside of your buttocks and the piriformis toward the middle of them.

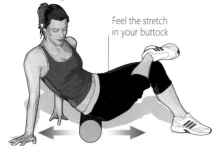

Feel the stretch in your buttock

1 Sit on the roller with your right buttock and cross your right leg over your left leg. Rolling backward and forward, work on the outside of your buttock before shifting your weight to the middle of your buttock. Repeat for at least 30 seconds before switching sides.

51 LAT FOAM ROLLER

This exercise helps loosen up the large muscles of your middle and upper back, reducing tightness.

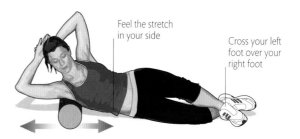

Feel the stretch in your side

Cross your left foot over your right foot

1 Lie on your right side over the roller, which should be placed under your armpit, and place your hands behind your head for stability. Use your back muscles to roll down from your armpit to the base of your shoulder blade. Roll back up and repeat for at least 30 seconds, then switch sides.

52 ITB FOAM ROLLER

This exercise loosens your iliotibial band (ITB), the band of muscular tissue on the outside of your upper leg, and can help prevent piriformis syndrome.

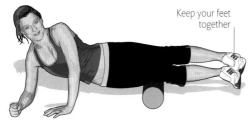

Keep your feet together

1 Lie on your right side with the foam roller beneath your outer thigh, just above your knee. Propping yourself up on your right forearm, bend your left arm slightly and place your left hand, palm-down, in front of you for support.

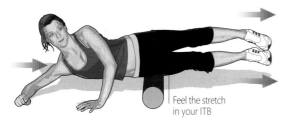

Feel the stretch in your ITB

2 Using your right forearm and left hand, push your body over the roller so that your outer thigh slides across the roller, up toward your hip bone. Slide back the opposite way and repeat for at least 30 seconds, then swap sides.

53 THORACIC FOAM ROLLER

Here, the foam roller acts as a hinge to help improve the range of motion in your middle and upper back. It is a good movement to help prevent neck and back pain.

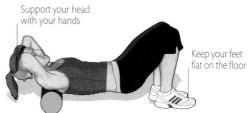

Support your head with your hands

Keep your feet flat on the floor

1 Sit with your heels planted on the floor and the roller beneath the middle of your back. Lie back onto the roller so that it is just below your shoulder blades. Clasp your hands together and lightly cradle your head.

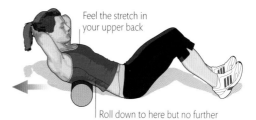

Feel the stretch in your upper back

Roll down to here but no further

2 With your chin tucked in, slide up and down the roller, from your neck down to the level of your lowest ribs. Do not go too low into your lumbar spine as this will cause some discomfort. Repeat for at least 30 seconds.

54 CURL-UP

A key part of most exercise programmes, this movement strengthens your abdominal muscles, which help to stabilize your pelvis. If it is recommended as part of your rehabilitation, you can increase the difficulty of the exercise through five levels as your strength and endurance gradually improve.

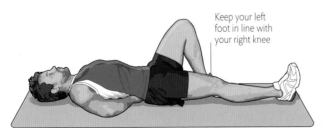

Keep your left foot in line with your right knee

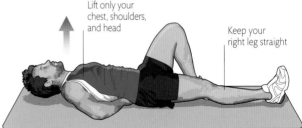

Lift only your chest, shoulders, and head

Keep your right leg straight

1 Lie on your back with one leg straight and the other bent at a 90-degree angle with your foot flat on the floor. Bend your elbows and place your hands palms-down under your lower back. Rest your elbows against the floor.

2 Use your stomach muscles to lift your chest, shoulders, and head off the floor, and breathe out. Hold for 8 seconds, then return to the start position for 2 seconds. Repeat as required, then switch leg positions.

PROGRESSION—LEVEL 2

Perform the curl-up as in Level 1, with your hands under the small of your back, but this time with your elbows off the floor. As for Level 1, keep one leg straight along the floor and the other bent at a right angle with your foot flat on the floor. Hold for 8 seconds at the top of the movement, then return to the start position for 2 seconds. Repeat as required, then switch leg positions.

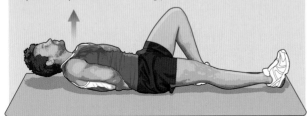

PROGRESSION—LEVEL 3

Place your hands across your chest instead of behind your back, straightening one leg along the floor and bending the other at 90 degrees with your foot flat on the floor, and only lift your chest, shoulders, and head off the floor. Hold for 8 seconds at the top, then return to the start position for 2 seconds. Repeat for the required number of reps, then switch leg positions.

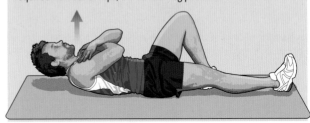

PROGRESSION—LEVEL 4

Position yourself with a wobble-board under your lower back and your hands across your chest, with one leg straight along the floor and the other bent at a right angle with your foot flat on the floor. Lift your chest, shoulders, and head, hold at the top for 8 seconds, then return to the start position for 2 seconds. Repeat for the required number of reps, then switch leg positions.

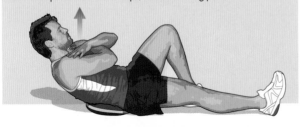

PROGRESSION—LEVEL 5

Perform the exercise with your lower back positioned on a Swiss ball and your hands across your chest. Plant your feet firmly on the floor and bend your knees at 90 degrees. Hold for 8 seconds, then return to the start position for 2 seconds. Repeat for the required number of reps.

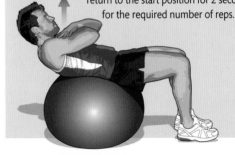

55 CAT AND CAMEL

A great muscle-releasing exercise, this stretch helps lubricate your spine and get your spinal discs moving. It is one of the best exercises you can do as part of a general warm-up.

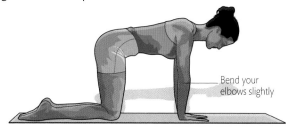

Bend your elbows slightly

1 Kneel on all fours with your hands in line with your shoulders, your fingers pointing forward, and your knees below your hips.

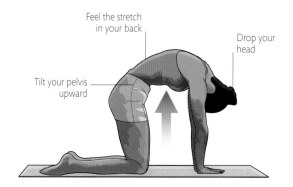

Feel the stretch in your back

Drop your head

Tilt your pelvis upward

2 Round your back upward and pull in your stomach, letting your head drop down. Pause at the top of the movement.

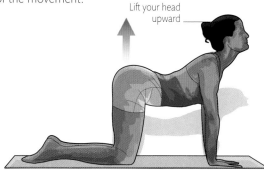

Lift your head upward

3 In one fluid movement, raise your buttocks and curve your spine downward while lifting your head so that you are looking straight ahead. Return to the start position and repeat as required.

56 SWISS BALL TWIST

This exercise not only helps build your abdominal muscles, but also strengthens the rotational muscles of your torso, improving your core stability and balance.

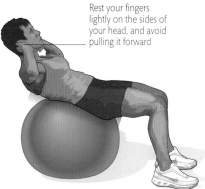

Rest your fingers lightly on the sides of your head, and avoid pulling it forward

1 Lie on a Swiss ball with your lower back supported, your feet flat on the floor, your knees at right angles, and your hands touching your head.

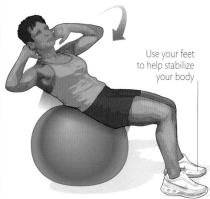

Use your feet to help stabilize your body

2 Once you feel steady, begin to crunch up. About halfway up, twist your torso to one side—spreading your elbows wide will help you to balance.

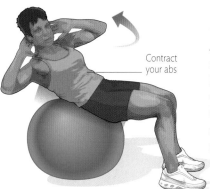

Contract your abs

3 Pause at the top of the movement, then lower and untwist your upper torso to return to the start position. Switch sides.

57 PLANK FROM KNEES

The plank is a simple move that trains your abdominals and spinal extensors as they work to maintain your raised position. You benefit from improved core strength, tighter abdominals, and a stronger back, all of which improve posture.

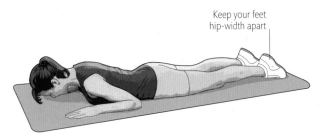

Keep your feet hip-width apart

1 Lie face down on a mat with your arms bent, elbows close to your sides, and palms facing down. Keep your head slightly raised off the floor.

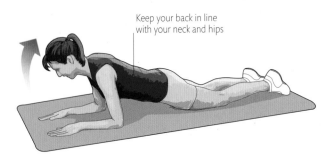

Keep your back in line with your neck and hips

2 Tighten your core and lift your abdomen, sliding your elbows forward directly under your shoulders to raise your hips off the floor and create a straight line from your knees to your shoulders. Keep your shoulder blades wide and apart, and your spine neutral. Hold this position for 15–20 seconds.

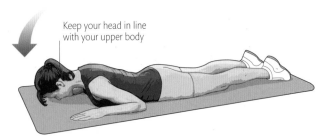

Keep your head in line with your upper body

3 Return to the start position and repeat 5 times, keeping your breathing regular throughout.

58 PRONE PLANK

This static floor exercise engages your core muscles, along with many of the major muscle groups of your upper and lower body, in order to maintain a fixed position. It can help to prevent lower-back problems or as part of your rehabilitation after a lower-back injury.

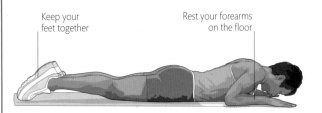

Keep your feet together

Rest your forearms on the floor

1 Lie face down on an exercise mat with your elbows to your sides and your hands alongside your head, palms facing the floor. Raise your head off the floor slightly. Rest the tips of your feet on the floor.

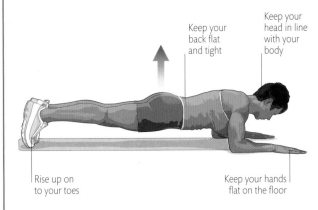

Keep your back flat and tight

Keep your head in line with your body

Rise up on to your toes

Keep your hands flat on the floor

2 Engaging your core and leg muscles, raise your body off the floor, supporting your weight on your forearms and toes, while breathing freely. Keep your head level. Hold the position for about 20 seconds.

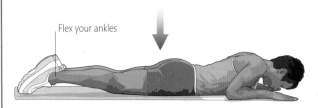

Flex your ankles

3 Gently lower your body back into the start position, and repeat as required.

59 SIDE PLANK (LEVEL 1)

This exercise works the muscles of your core, which support your spine. It is key in the rehabilitation of any injury to either your back or pelvis. The most basic form of this exercise is good for initial rehabilitation, and is a starting point for those who have not done it before or do not have sufficient core stability.

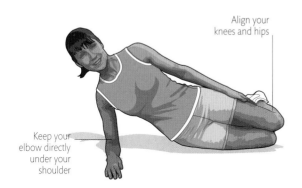

Align your knees and hips

Keep your elbow directly under your shoulder

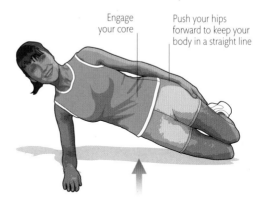

Engage your core

Push your hips forward to keep your body in a straight line

1 Lying on your right side, prop yourself up on your right forearm and bend your knees so that your calves are at a right angle. Make sure that your right elbow is directly under your shoulder and in line with your hips. Rest your left arm along the side of your body.

2 Engage your abdominals and push down through your right elbow to raise your hips off the floor, making sure that you keep your rib cage elevated and your shoulder lowered. Hold for 8 seconds, then return to the start position for 2 seconds. Repeat as required, then switch sides.

60 SIDE PLANK (LEVEL 2)

This progression of the basic side plank exercise (»above) makes the muscles of your core work harder, as you are using them to stabilize your body, while supporting your weight on your arm and ankles.

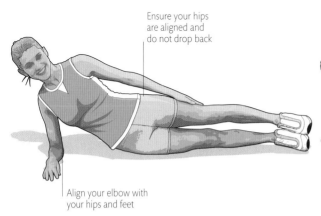

Ensure your hips are aligned and do not drop back

Align your elbow with your hips and feet

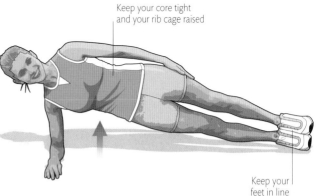

Keep your core tight and your rib cage raised

Keep your feet in line

1 Lying on your right side, prop yourself up on your right forearm. Extend your legs and keep your feet together. Make sure that your right elbow is directly under your shoulder and in line with your hips. Rest your left arm along your side.

2 Engage your abdominals and push downward through your right elbow to raise your hips off the ground, ensuring you keep your ribcage elevated and your shoulder lowered. Hold for 8 seconds, then return to the start position for 2 seconds. Repeat as required, then switch sides.

61 **SWISS BALL** SIDE CRUNCH

This exercise improves your strength, core stability, and balance. It is quite advanced, so you should perform it under guidance, and only once you have mastered curl-ups on the ball (»p.94) and side crunches (»p.119).

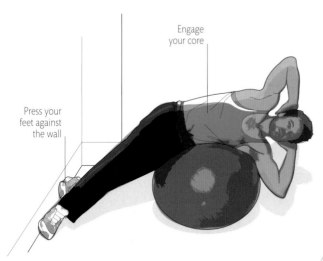

Engage your core

Press your feet against the wall

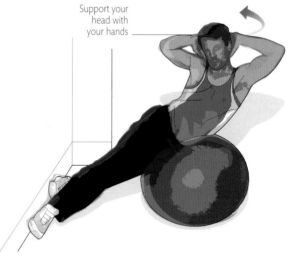

Support your head with your hands

1 Rest your left hip and side on a Swiss ball, pressing your feet against the wall for support, with your right leg in front of your left. Bend your arms at the elbows, with your hands touching the sides of your head.

2 Slowly raise your torso up to your right side, keeping the ball as still as possible by using the wall as a support. Hold this position for 2–3 seconds, then return to the start position. Repeat 10 times, then switch sides.

62 **SWISS BALL** SIDE CRUNCH WITH TWIST

This is an advanced exercise designed to improve strength, core stability, and balance. Perform it under guidance once you've mastered the easier exercises such as side crunches (»p.119), and curl-ups on the ball (»p.94).

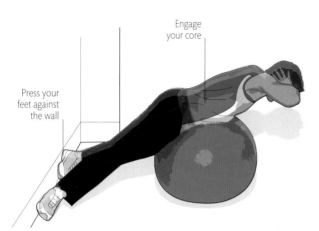

Engage your core

Press your feet against the wall

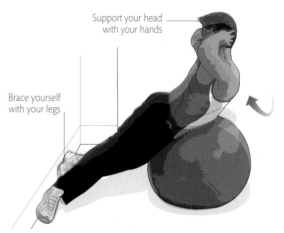

Support your head with your hands

Brace yourself with your legs

1 Rest your left hip and pelvis on a Swiss ball with your chest facing the ground and your arms bent at the elbows, hands touching the sides of your head. Press your feet against the wall for support, with your right leg in front of your left.

2 Slowly lift your torso while rotating your trunk to the right, so that your chest faces the wall. Hold this position for 2–3 seconds, then return to start position. Repeat 10 times, then switch sides.

63 KNEELING SUPERMAN

This exercise strengthens the spinal extensor muscles and deep spinal stabilizers, which support your spine, and builds strength and stability in your core, lower back, and shoulders. It is a key movement for maintaining a healthy back, and an important rehabilitation exercise for a number of back conditions.

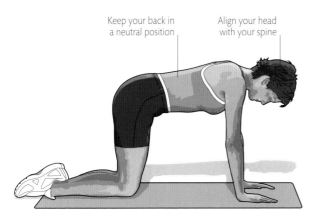

Keep your back in a neutral position

Align your head with your spine

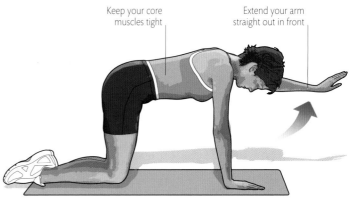

Keep your core muscles tight

Extend your arm straight out in front

1 Kneel on all fours, ensuring that your knees are aligned squarely under your hips. Keep your back straight and position your hands directly beneath your shoulders, pressing them flat on the ground and pointing forward.

2 Engaging your core, raise one arm in front of you. Hold for 10 seconds and return to the start position. Repeat with your other arm.

PROGRESSION—LEVEL 2

Raising a leg rather than an arm will demand more balance and control. Engage your abdominal muscles and lift your right leg behind you to hip height. Balance and hold for 10 seconds, then return to the start position. Be careful to keep your back straight and avoid arching your spine. Repeat with your other leg.

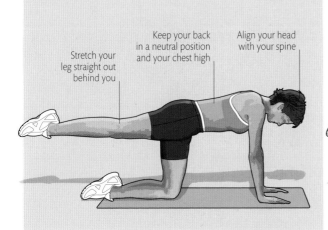

Stretch your leg straight out behind you

Keep your back in a neutral position and your chest high

Align your head with your spine

PROGRESSION—LEVEL 3

Combining an arm lift and a leg lift requires good strength and stability. Contracting your abs, simultaneously lift your right leg behind you to hip height and your left arm forward to shoulder height. Hold for 10 seconds, then lower your leg and arm to the start position with control. Keep your body straight, and repeat with your other leg and arm.

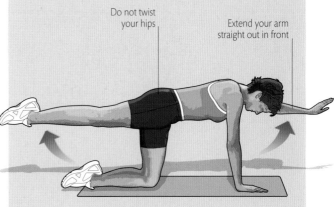

Do not twist your hips

Extend your arm straight out in front

64 MCKENZIE EXTENSION

This exercise helps to ease aches in your lower back, such as those caused by sitting for long periods of time. It is sometimes helpful in reducing pain if you have been diagnosed with a herniated disk or disk-related sciatica. You may feel some discomfort, but stop if you feel pain. Aim to perform 10 reps, several times a day.

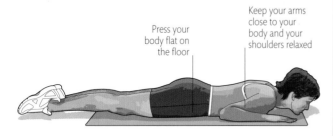

Press your body flat on the floor

Keep your arms close to your body and your shoulders relaxed

1 Lie face down on a mat with your hands flat on the floor and roughly level with your chin. Extend your feet, keeping your legs together.

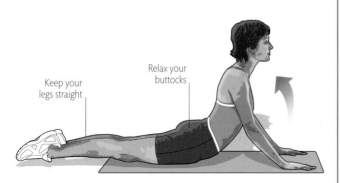

Keep your legs straight

Relax your buttocks

2 Pressing your hips against the mat and exhaling, lift your torso upward slowly, using your arms for support. Raise your head and shoulders up as high as you can, keeping your lower back relaxed. Pause briefly at the top of the movement and use your arms to lower your torso back to the start position.

VARIATION

If your injury means that one side of your back is more painful than the other, there is a useful variation of this exercise. While you are lying face-down on your stomach, as in Step 1, shift your legs toward your painful side before you extend your upper torso upward.

65 LEG RAISE

This exercise strengthens your hip flexors and your core, and is a useful movement to help stabilize your pelvis and prevent lower-back problems. Ensure you use the muscles of your core and legs, rather than your back.

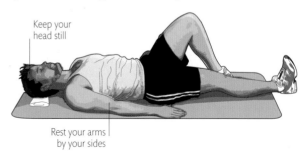

Keep your head still

Rest your arms by your sides

1 Lie on your back with your head on a folded towel. Bend your left knee to relax your lower back, with your arms by your sides, hands palms-down, and your right foot pointing upward.

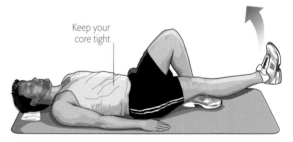

Keep your core tight

2 Keeping your knee straight, lift your right leg about 16 in (40 cm) off the floor (or higher as your muscles grow stronger) in a slow, fluid movement.

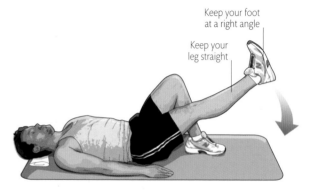

Keep your foot at a right angle

Keep your leg straight

3 Pause at the top of the movement for 3–5 seconds, then return to the start position, slowly and under control. Perform 15 reps, then switch legs.

66 **SIDE-LYING LEG** RAISE

This exercise strengthens your gluteus medius muscles in your buttocks, which play a key role in pelvic stability and in the prevention of back problems. Use your core and leg muscles rather than your back.

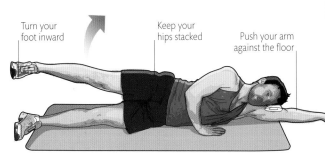

Lie with your hips, knees, and feet stacked

Extend your arm above your head for support

1 Lie on your left side and stretch your left arm out, so that your legs, body, and head are aligned. Place a towel between your head and arm to help keep your upper body relaxed, and use your upper arms to support you and stop you rolling forward and backward.

Turn your foot inward

Keep your hips stacked

Push your arm against the floor

2 Keeping your knee straight and your foot turned inward to maximize the benefit of the movement, lift your right leg about 16 in (40 cm) off the floor. Ensure you keep your core engaged to prevent lower-back strain.

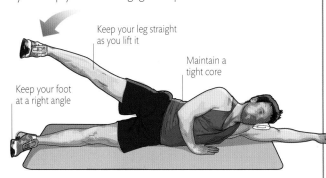

Keep your leg straight as you lift it

Maintain a tight core

Keep your foot at a right angle

3 Pausing at the top of the movement for about 3–5 seconds, return to the start position, slowly and with control. Perform 15 reps, then switch legs.

67 **REVERSE LEG** RAISE

This exercise strengthens the gluteus maximus muscles in your buttocks. It promotes good pelvic stability and helps in the prevention and rehabilitation of lower-back problems. If your buttock muscles are weak, you may be tempted to use your back in the movement. You can prevent this by placing a pillow under your abdomen and pelvis.

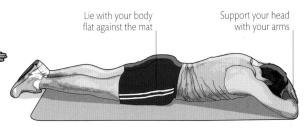

Lie with your body flat against the mat

Support your head with your arms

1 Lie on your front with your forehead resting on the back of your hands and your knees straight. Brace your abdomen and squeeze your buttocks tightly together.

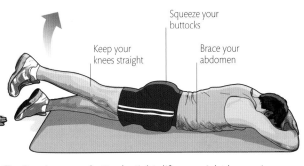

Squeeze your buttocks

Keep your knees straight

Brace your abdomen

2 Keeping your buttocks tight, lift your right leg up in a slow, fluid movement about 12 in (30 cm) off the floor (or higher as your muscles grow stronger).

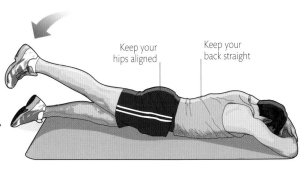

Keep your hips aligned

Keep your back straight

3 Pause for 3–5 seconds when you reach the top of the movement, then return to the start position, slowly and with control. Perform 15 reps, then switch legs.

68 ISOMETRIC ADDUCTOR SQUEEZE

This is a key exercise for the rehabilitation of sacroiliac joint dysfunction because regaining strength in your adductor muscles is essential for the treatment and prevention of lower-back pain.

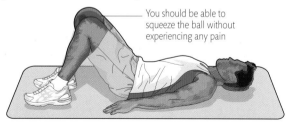

You should be able to squeeze the ball without experiencing any pain

1 Lie on your back with your pelvis in a neutral position, knees bent at a right angle, and feet flat on the floor. Place a medicine ball between your knees. Squeeze as hard as is comfortable, hold for 10 seconds, and relax to return to the start position. Repeat the movement as required.

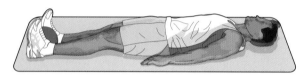

2 Place a medicine ball between your ankles. Lie on your back with your pelvis in a neutral position and keep your legs straight. Squeeze the ball between your ankles as hard as you can, hold for 10 seconds, and return to the start position. Repeat as required. This movement should not be painful.

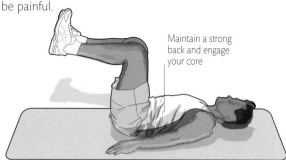

Maintain a strong back and engage your core

3 Lie on your back with your pelvis in a neutral position, and your hips and knees bent at right angles. Place a medicine ball between your knees. Squeeze as hard as is comfortable, hold for 10 seconds, then relax to the start position. Perform the necessary number of repetitions. You should not experience any pain when you squeeze the ball.

69 ADDUCTOR LIFT

This is a great exercise for strengthening your adductors. Weak adductors can lead to poor hip position and sacroiliac joint dysfunction. As your strength increases, you can use ankle weights to make it harder.

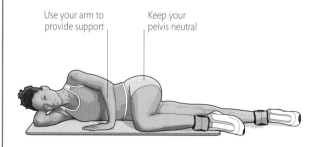

Use your arm to provide support

Keep your pelvis neutral

1 Lie on your right side with your hips stacked and your right arm bent under your head. Shift your weight forward, using your left arm for balance. Bend your left leg to 90 degrees, with your left knee touching the floor. Keep your right leg straight. Breathe in.

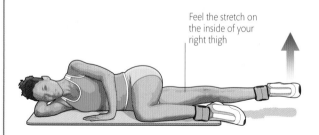

Feel the stretch on the inside of your right thigh

2 Keeping your arms and left leg in the same position, raise your right leg off the ground as high as you can, exhaling as you lift, then pause.

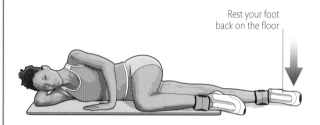

Rest your foot back on the floor

3 Return to the start position, inhaling as you lower your leg. Repeat as necessary, before switching sides to work your left leg.

70 BRIDGE

This exercise activates the large gluteal muscles of your buttocks and your hamstrings. It is an important core-stabilizing movement for the rehabilitation of numerous back problems, including sacroiliac joint pain. There is a wide range of potential variations, making it a very versatile exercise. As your strength increases, you can try the single-leg bridge (»below).

VARIATION

This exercise can be varied by bending your knees further, or putting your feet on a Swiss ball. This adds a level of instability, making your core stabilizers work harder.

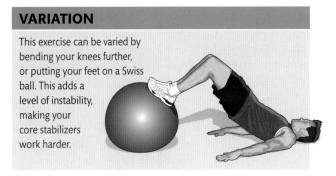

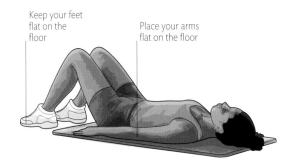

Keep your feet flat on the floor

Place your arms flat on the floor

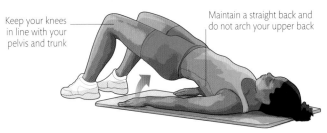

Keep your knees in line with your pelvis and trunk

Maintain a straight back and do not arch your upper back

1 Lie on your back with your knees bent at right angles and your feet flat on the floor, hip-width apart. Keep your arms at your sides, with your palms facing down.

2 Engaging your core, slowly lift your buttocks off the floor until your body is in a straight line from your knees to your shoulders. Pause at the top, then reverse the movement to return to the starting position.

71 SINGLE-LEG BRIDGE

A development of the bridge (»above), this exercise is useful for working the large gluteal muscles of your buttocks, your hip extensors, and your core. Because you are performing it on one leg, it forces you to control the rotation and tilt of your pelvis. It is important to ensure that you keep your hips level throughout.

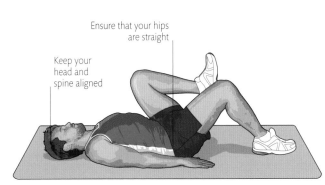

Ensure that your hips are straight

Keep your head and spine aligned

Keep your hips fixed and do not twist

Engage your abdominals

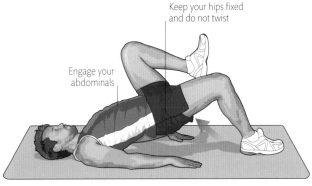

1 Lie on your back with your knees bent at 90 degrees, your feet hip-width apart, and your hands palms-down by your sides. Keeping your right foot flat on the floor, and your arms by your sides, raise your left knee up toward your torso until your thighs are at right angles.

2 Engaging the muscles of your abdomen and lower back, lift your buttocks until your hips are fully extended and your body is in a straight line from your lower knee to your shoulders. Hold this position, then reverse the movement to return to the start position, and switch legs.

72 LAT STRETCH

Specifically targeting the large muscles of your upper back, this simple stretch is a useful exercise for maintenance and rehabilitation for a range of back injuries.

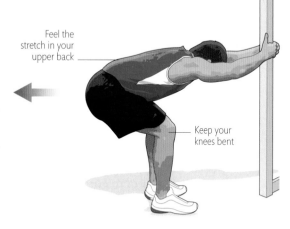

Feel the stretch in your upper back

Keep your knees bent

1 Stand facing an upright support that will take your weight. Grip the support with both hands and lean back, bending your knees. Push with your legs and pull with your arms.

73 QUAD STRETCH

This stretch works the quadriceps muscles at the front of your thigh, which enable you to straighten your knee. Because this stretch is performed in a standing position, it emphasizes good posture and balance.

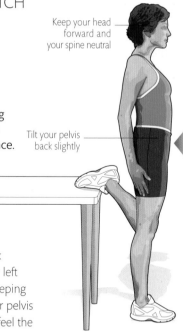

Keep your head forward and your spine neutral

Tilt your pelvis back slightly

1 Stand with your back to a table. Place your left foot on the table and, keeping your legs parallel, tilt your pelvis back slightly so you can feel the stretch in the front of your left thigh. Hold, lower, and repeat with your right leg.

74 HAMSTRING STRETCH 1

This is a simple general-purpose stretch that works all the muscles in your hamstrings, relieving the tightness that can stress your lower back. Stretch slowly and avoid "bouncing" at full extension.

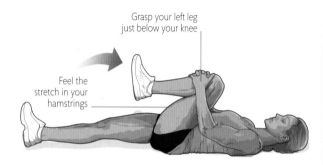

Grasp your left leg just below your knee

Feel the stretch in your hamstrings

1 Lie on your back with your legs extended. Bend your left knee. Pull gently on your left leg, bringing your knee toward your chest until you feel the stretch. Keep the back of your head on the floor. Relax and repeat with your right leg.

75 HAMSTRING STRETCH 2

This is another useful stretch for your hamstring muscles to help relieve tightness, which can cause pain in your lower back. Perform the stretch in a slow, controlled manner.

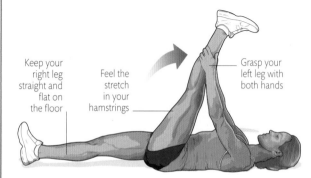

Keep your right leg straight and flat on the floor

Feel the stretch in your hamstrings

Grasp your left leg with both hands

1 Lie on your back with your legs extended. Lift each leg in turn, keeping your knee braced and your toes pulled back toward your body. If you are very flexible, try extending the stretch a little by pulling back on your leg.

76 LANCELOT STRETCH

This is a useful stretch if you suffer from stiffness around your spine, as it stretches your hip flexors and, in particular, your psoas muscle. Your psoas muscle is directly attached to your spine and it is important to keep it flexible.

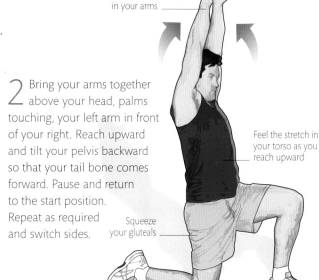

Look straight ahead

Bend your leg so that your knee is at a right angle

Feel the stretch in your arms

Feel the stretch in your torso as you reach upward

Squeeze your gluteals

1 Stand with your feet shoulder-width apart and your hands on your hips. Lunge forward with your left leg, bending both legs so that your right knee and the top of your right foot are touching the floor. Keep your spine neutral and look straight ahead.

2 Bring your arms together above your head, palms touching, your left arm in front of your right. Reach upward and tilt your pelvis backward so that your tail bone comes forward. Pause and return to the start position. Repeat as required and switch sides.

77 ADDUCTOR STRETCH 1

Stretching your adductor or groin muscles is key to maintaining hip flexibility, and can help with lower-back pain.

Keep your body upright

Feel the stretch in your adductors

1 Keep your body upright and put your hands on your hips. Bend your left leg so that your left knee is over your left foot, your right leg is extended, and your right foot is flat. Rock gently to the side. Relax and switch legs.

78 ADDUCTOR STRETCH 2

This version of the adductor stretch works more on the short adductor muscles of your groin. It is easy to perform, can be carried out almost anywhere, and forms a useful part of a general stretching routine.

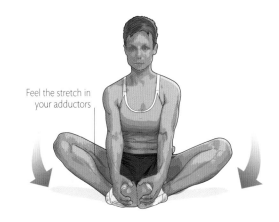

Feel the stretch in your adductors

1 Sit on the floor and take a firm hold of the tops of your feet. Bring your legs in close to your body, pressing the soles of your feet together. Push your knees gently down toward the floor as far as you can, and hold.

79 PIRIFORMIS STRETCH

This seated stretch is more advanced than the ITB foam roller stretch (»p.93) because you need greater flexibility in your hip joint to perform it correctly. It is useful for preventing or easing piriformis syndrome, and is particularly important for those who exercise regularly.

1 Sit on the floor with your legs extended. Support yourself with your left hand behind you, and bend your left leg, crossing it over your right leg. Keep your left foot flat on the floor. Reach over with your right hand and gently press on the outside of your left knee until you can feel the stretch in the outside of your thigh. Hold briefly, then switch sides.

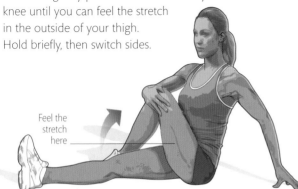

Feel the stretch here

80 CALF STRETCH

Tight calf muscles can cause a muscular imbalance by making your foot turn outward and forcing your hip muscles to work harder. Your gait may become "flatter," which can lead to back pain.

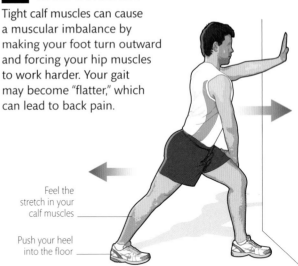

Feel the stretch in your calf muscles

Push your heel into the floor

1 From a standing position, press your left hand against a wall and take a good step backward with your right leg, keeping your feet hip-width apart. Bend your left leg forward, ensuring you keep your knee over your foot. Switch arms and repeat with your other leg.

81 CALF RAISE

This exercise helps to strengthen your calf muscles and improve your gait. It is important to avoid tight calf muscles, as they can put stress on the muscles of your lower back, and cause or aggravate pain in that area.

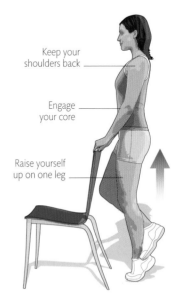

Keep your supporting leg straight

Keep your shoulders back

Engage your core

Raise yourself up on one leg

1 Stand on your left leg, with the toe of your right leg wrapped around the back of your left ankle. Support your body weight with your left leg, and rest your hands on the back of a chair. Inhale.

2 Raise yourself up as high as you can go onto the ball of your left foot, exhaling as you do so. Pause briefly, then lower your heel back to the start position, breathing in. Repeat as required, then switch legs.

82 SINGLE-LEG STAND

This exercise is a good starting point for developing your balance in a weight-bearing position. It also improves control of your trunk and strengthens your buttock muscles, helping improve your pelvic stability.

1 Pick a point on the wall in front of you and focus on it. Stand on one leg and tighten your buttocks and thighs all at the same time. Stand in front of a mirror if you need to check that your posture and form are correct.

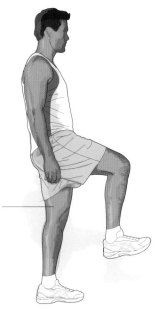

Contract the muscles in the buttock and thigh of your standing leg

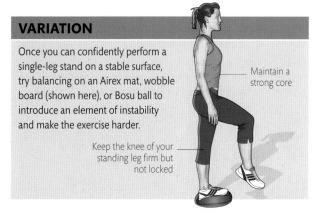

VARIATION

Once you can confidently perform a single-leg stand on a stable surface, try balancing on an Airex mat, wobble board (shown here), or Bosu ball to introduce an element of instability and make the exercise harder.

Maintain a strong core

Keep the knee of your standing leg firm but not locked

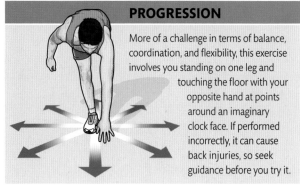

PROGRESSION

More of a challenge in terms of balance, coordination, and flexibility, this exercise involves you standing on one leg and touching the floor with your opposite hand at points around an imaginary clock face. If performed incorrectly, it can cause back injuries, so seek guidance before you try it.

83 WALL-SUPPORTED FOOT LIFT

This exercise strengthens the muscles of your feet and lower legs. It helps prevent flat feet and overpronation (»p.37), and improves your gait. It can help to prevent problems in your knees, hip, and back in the longer term.

1 Rest your head, shoulders, back, and arms against a wall. Move your feet slightly apart and 12 in (30 cm) from the wall, bending your knees slightly.

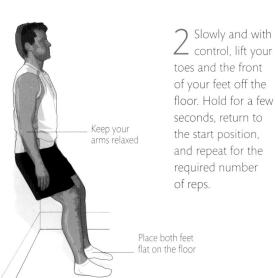

Keep your arms relaxed

Place both feet flat on the floor

2 Slowly and with control, lift your toes and the front of your feet off the floor. Hold for a few seconds, return to the start position, and repeat for the required number of reps.

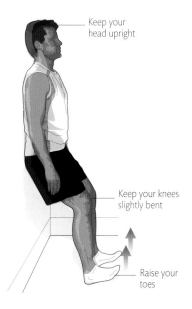

Keep your head upright

Keep your knees slightly bent

Raise your toes

84 SUPINE PELVIC TILT

This exercise helps with most types of acute lumbar pain by relieving pressure on the facet joints and gently stretching the muscles and ligaments of your back, strengthening your core and improving your posture. You should perform this exercise on the floor at first, but as you improve you can try it standing up.

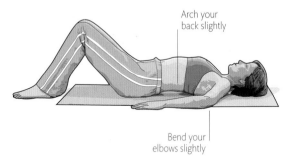

Arch your back slightly

Bend your elbows slightly

1 Lie on your back with your knees bent at a comfortable angle, your feet flat on the floor, your arms by your sides at a slight bend, and your lower back arched but relaxed.

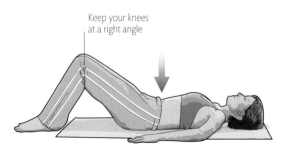

Keep your knees at a right angle

2 Gently press the small of your back into the floor and tilt your pubic bone upward by tightening your abdominal and pelvic floor muscles. Hold for at least 6 seconds.

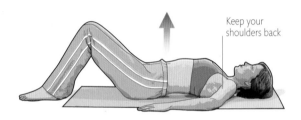

Keep your shoulders back

3 Relax and return to the start position, so that the small of your back is slightly arched once more. Repeat as required and relax.

85 KNEELING PELVIC TILT

This exercise helps those with poor posture. Some experts recommend this as an alternative for the supine version of the exercise (»left) after the first trimester of pregnancy because that version may interfere with blood supply to the fetus.

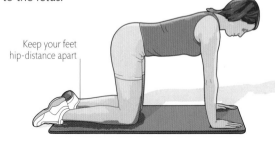

Keep your feet hip-distance apart

1 Kneel on a mat with your hands under your shoulders and your knees under your hips, keeping your back in a neutral position, and breathe in deeply.

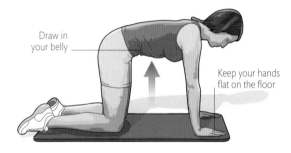

Draw in your belly

Keep your hands flat on the floor

2 Breathe out, pulling your abdominals in tight, and suck in your belly button toward your spine. With one fluid motion, reverse the curve in your lower back and tilt your hips.

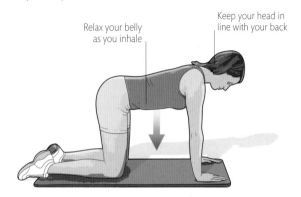

Relax your belly as you inhale

Keep your head in line with your back

3 Release and repeat for the required number of reps. Inhale and exhale as you perform the moves, feeling the pull and push of the movement deep within your core.

86 SEATED PELVIC TILT

It is harder to perform the pelvic tilt in an upright posture, either standing or sitting, but doing this exercise on a Swiss ball provides a helpful guide, as the ball will shift forward slightly when you do the movement correctly.

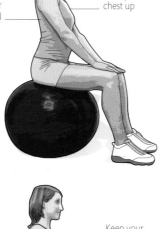

Keep your back straight and your spine neutral

Hold your chest up

1 Sit up straight on a Swiss ball, with your feet parallel and hip-width apart. Rest your hands on your knees. Keep your back straight and your spine neutral. Breathe in deeply and arch your back slightly.

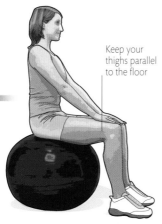

Keep your thighs parallel to the floor

2 Exhale forcefully, pulling your abdominals in tight and drawing them in toward your spine. With one fluid motion, reverse the curve in your lower back by tucking your hips under your torso and rolling the ball forward very slightly as you do so.

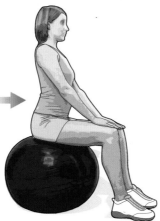

3 Hold the position for a few seconds, then release to return to the arched position in Step 1. Repeat as required and relax.

87 PRONE BACK EXTENSION

This is a good maintenance exercise for the muscles of your lower back and core, but you should only attempt it if your lower back is free of pain. The only sensation you should feel while performing it is the muscles of your lower back tightening as they work.

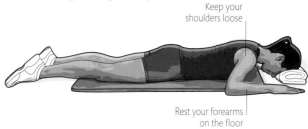

Keep your shoulders loose

Rest your forearms on the floor

1 Lie face down on a mat with a folded towel under your forehead to ensure proper alignment of your head and neck with your spine. Bend your arms and rest your forearms on the floor, palms down. Inhale deeply.

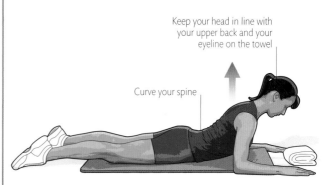

Keep your head in line with your upper back and your eyeline on the towel

Curve your spine

2 Engage your core and reach forward with the top of your head to lengthen your spine, keeping your shoulders apart. Then, facing downward, lift your head and shoulders off the floor, exhaling as you do so. Make sure that you do not use any strength from your arms.

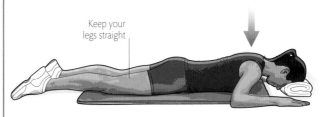

Keep your legs straight

3 Pause at the top of the movement, then inhale and slowly return to the start position without resting. Repeat as required.

88 STANDING BACK EXTENSION

This exercise gently arches your lower back, and it is useful for lumbar disk problems. You should perform it every couple of hours through the day. If it increases your pain, try the prone back extension exercise (»p.109) instead.

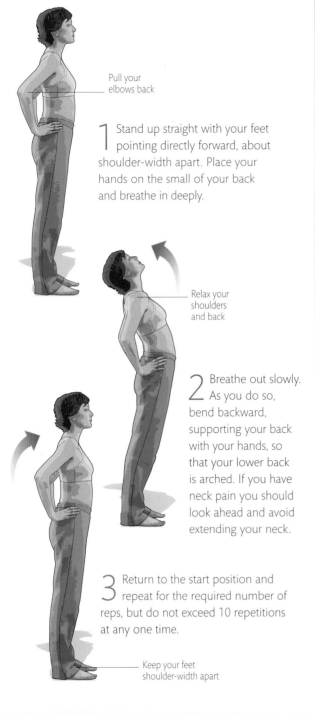

Pull your elbows back

1 Stand up straight with your feet pointing directly forward, about shoulder-width apart. Place your hands on the small of your back and breathe in deeply.

Relax your shoulders and back

2 Breathe out slowly. As you do so, bend backward, supporting your back with your hands, so that your lower back is arched. If you have neck pain you should look ahead and avoid extending your neck.

3 Return to the start position and repeat for the required number of reps, but do not exceed 10 repetitions at any one time.

Keep your feet shoulder-width apart

89 KNEES-TO-CHEST STRETCH

This exercise helps if you have strained a facet joint, and the surrounding muscles are tight and aching. However, you should proceed with caution if you know your pain is caused by a disk protrusion.

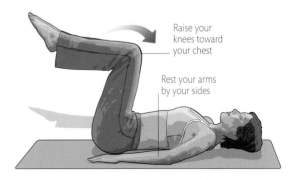

Raise your knees toward your chest

Rest your arms by your sides

1 Lie down and do a basic pelvic tilt (»p.108). Then draw your knees up toward your chest, keeping your lower back flat.

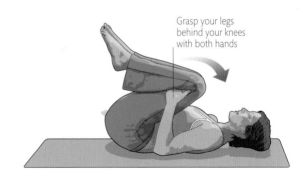

Grasp your legs behind your knees with both hands

2 Use your hands to help draw your knees closer to your chest. Keep your head on the floor.

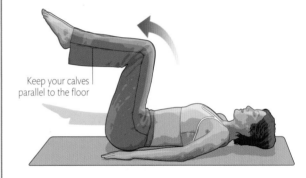

Keep your calves parallel to the floor

3 Let go of your thighs and return to the start position. Repeat for the required number of reps.

90 **SWISS BALL** BACK EXTENSION

This advanced exercise requires you to stabilize the full length of your body while increasing resistance (by placing your hands behind your head) and range of motion (the ball adds height to the lift).

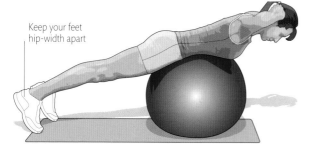

Keep your feet hip-width apart

1 Position your torso on a Swiss ball with your legs extended, and dig your toes into the mat. Alternatively, plant your feet against a wall. Rest your fingertips lightly at the back of your head and lengthen your spine. Breathe in.

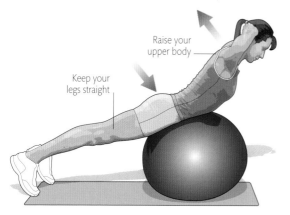

Raise your upper body

Keep your legs straight

2 Exhale as you squeeze your buttocks and slowly lift your torso to 45 degrees. Press your hips into the ball. Pause at the top, then inhale.

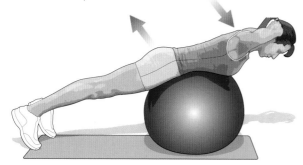

3 Slowly return to the start position without resting. Gradually build up the number of reps.

91 **BACK** ROTATION

This exercise improves general mobility and is particularly useful for relaxing the muscles of your back and pelvis. It also relieves facet joint pain by stretching the capsules and ligaments around the facet joints in your lower back: those on your left will be stretched as you drop your knees to the right, and vice versa.

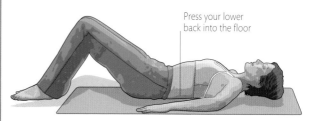

Press your lower back into the floor

1 Lie on your back with your knees bent, your feet flat on the floor and your arms by your sides, as for the pelvic tilt (»p.108). Press your lower back into the floor.

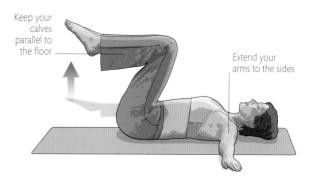

Keep your calves parallel to the floor

Extend your arms to the sides

2 Keeping your knees together, lift them until they are above the middle of your abdominal region, and bring your arms straight out to your sides.

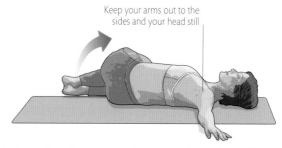

Keep your arms out to the sides and your head still

3 Let your legs flop over to the right as far as they will go. Breathe slowly and deeply, allowing your legs to drop a little farther with each breath. Hold for as long as you can, then bring your legs back up and lower them to the other side. Repeat the movement as required.

92 FOUR-POINT SUPINE KNEE LIFT

This is a moderate-impact core-stabilizing exercise. It can be helpful for strengthening the deep muscles of your abdomen and your lower back, and can be a useful exercise for preventing pain in your lumbar region. To get the best results from the movement, keep the muscles of your core engaged throughout.

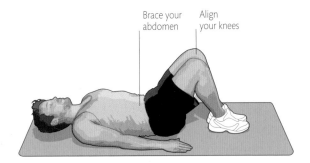

Brace your abdomen

Align your knees

1 Lie on your back and bend your knees, with your feet flat on the floor. Relax your shoulders and upper back, brace your abdomen, and keep your spine in a neutral position.

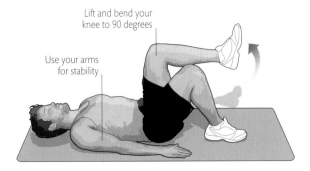

Lift and bend your knee to 90 degrees

Use your arms for stability

2 Keeping your abdomen braced, lift your left leg so that your hip and knee are at right angles. Keep your right foot firmly on the floor.

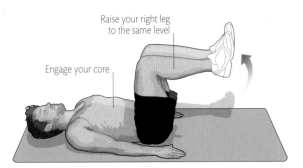

Raise your right leg to the same level

Engage your core

3 Still keeping your abdomen braced, lift your right leg until it is level with your left. Hold this position for a few seconds and use your arms to stabilize yourself.

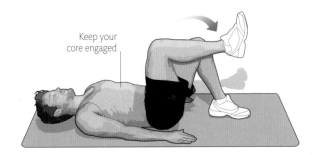

Keep your core engaged

4 Keeping your core engaged, slowly lower your left leg until your foot is flat on the floor.

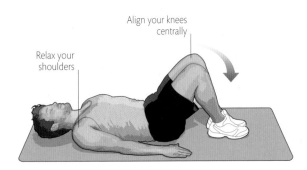

Align your knees centrally

Relax your shoulders

5 Now lower your right leg, returning to the start position. Repeat the exercise 5 times and then repeat the sequence beginning with your right leg.

VARIATION

Once you can perform the basic four-point supine knee lift with confidence and you have improved the strength and stability in your abdomen and lumbar region, you can make the exercise harder by placing an air cushion (shown here) or Bosu board in the small of your back. Focus on maintaining stability in your torso and keeping the muscles of your core engaged. Try not to use your arms to keep you balanced.

Position the air cushion beneath your pelvis

93 ISOMETRIC HIP FLEXION

This exercise strengthens your deep abdominal muscles and hip flexors, and stabilizes your lower back. It can be used to treat sacroiliac joint dysfunction and lumbar hypermobility.

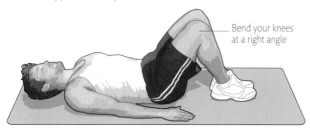

Bend your knees at a right angle

1 Lie on your back and bend your knees. Relax your shoulders and upper back, brace your abdomen, and keep your spine in a neutral position.

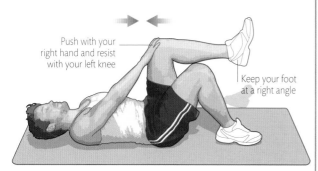

Push with your right hand and resist with your left knee

Keep your foot at a right angle

2 Place your right hand on your left knee. Push your knee and flex your hip simultaneously: the force of the push and flexion of the hip should be equal, so no movement will occur. Hold for 10 seconds.

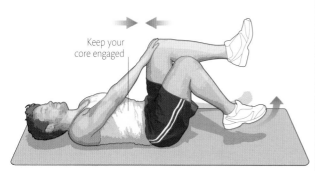

Keep your core engaged

3 Maintaining the resistance between your left knee and right hand, raise your right foot off the mat. Hold for 5 seconds, then relax and return to the start position. Perform the move 5 times, then change legs.

94 SINGLE-LEG ELONGATION

This exercise is used in the rehabilitation of facet joint and sacroiliac joint dysfunction; it also stretches the muscles of your lower back, and can help with three-curve scoliosis. Perform this exercise only on the affected side.

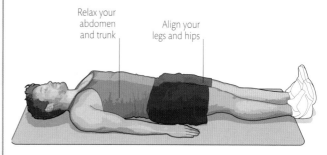

Relax your abdomen and trunk

Align your legs and hips

1 Lie on your back with your feet hip-width apart and your arms by your sides, palms down.

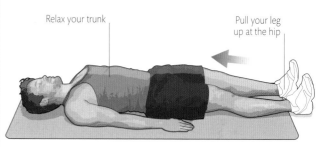

Relax your trunk

Pull your leg up at the hip

2 Keeping your arms by your sides, pull your unaffected leg up at the hip to shorten it.

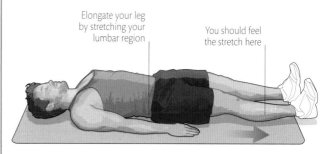

Elongate your leg by stretching your lumbar region

You should feel the stretch here

3 Now elongate the leg on your affected side by stretching the side of your lower back and your hip joint. Hold the position for 5 seconds, then relax. Repeat for 3 sets of 5 reps, only on this affected side.

95 PRONE KNEE BEND

This exercise is used to mobilize the femoral nerve and stretch tight muscles at the front of your hip and thigh. It can be useful for increasing the range of motion in damaged knee joints, and helps to prevent lower-back pain.

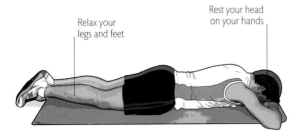

Relax your legs and feet

Rest your head on your hands

1 Lie face down on a mat. Bend your arms in front of you and rest your forehead on your hands. Relax your trunk and legs.

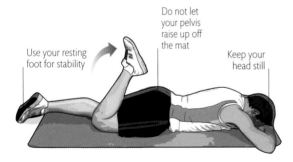

Do not let your pelvis raise up off the mat

Use your resting foot for stability

Keep your head still

2 Keeping your left leg flat on the mat, bend your right leg up as far as you can in a slow, relaxed motion. Ensure that you keep your hips still as you perform the movement.

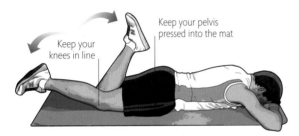

Keep your pelvis pressed into the mat

Keep your knees in line

3 Lower your right leg down and bend your left leg up simultaneously. Continue alternating legs, repeating 10 times for each leg, slowly and under control, then return to the start position.

96 SIDE GLIDE

This exercise was developed by physical therapist Robin McKenzie to alleviate acute lower-back pain due to disk problems that have shifted the pelvis to one side. Look in a mirror: if your right hip is more prominent, this exercise should help you pull your pelvis to the left and glide your trunk to the right. If your left hip is more prominent, do the exercise the other way around.

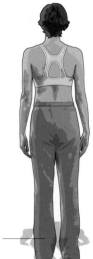

1 Stand with your feet shoulder-width apart, knees straight and arms hanging loosely beside you.

Relax your arms

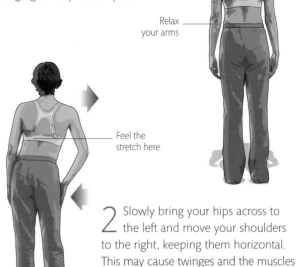

Feel the stretch here

2 Slowly bring your hips across to the left and move your shoulders to the right, keeping them horizontal. This may cause twinges and the muscles will tighten up in resistance. Stop if the pain increases in your back or legs.

3 Relax and return to the start position. Repeat the sequence until you return to a neutral position with no lateral shift. Repeat 10 times every 2 hours. Once your tilt is corrected you can start prone (»p.109) or standing back extensions (»p.110).

Keep your legs straight and shoulder-width apart

97 STATIONARY LUNGE

Lunges are fantastic exercises for your buttocks and thighs, and can help prevent lower-back problems, as these muscles provide support to your back. Though you will feel the front of your thigh working first, the lunge is also strengthening your buttocks and the backs of your thighs, and helping to improve your hip mobility.

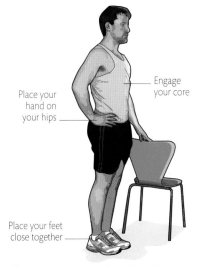

Place your hand on your hips

Engage your core

Place your feet close together

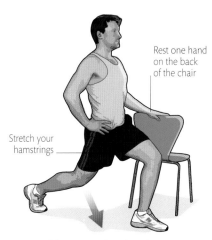

Rest one hand on the back of the chair

Stretch your hamstrings

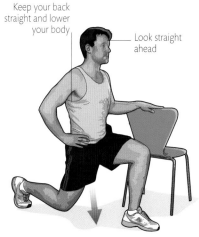

Keep your back straight and lower your body

Look straight ahead

1 Stand with your feet slightly apart, your right hand on your hip, and your left hand resting on a chair back. Align your shoulders, hips, and feet.

2 Holding onto the chair, bring your left leg back, heel lifted, keeping your legs parallel. Keep your hips facing forward and your weight centered evenly.

3 Inhale and lower your right knee, with your left knee over your ankle. Exhale as you straighten your legs. Repeat as required, then switch sides.

98 FORWARD LUNGE

Once you are comfortable with the stationary lunge (**»above**), you can progress to this unsupported version of the exercise. This version of the lunge requires more balance as you do not have a chair to hold onto.

1 Stand with your feet hip-width apart and your hands on your hips. Keep your shoulders, hips, and feet in line.

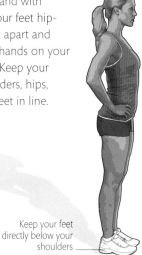

Keep your feet directly below your shoulders

2 Step forward with your right leg and come up on the toes of your left foot. Bend both knees so that your right knee is bent above your ankle and your left knee is close to the floor.

Look straight ahead

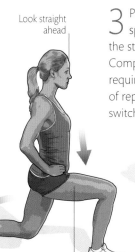

Lunge forward

3 Pause, then spring back to the start position. Complete the required number of reps, then switch legs.

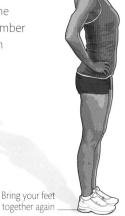

Bring your feet together again

99 REVERSE LUNGE WITH KNEE LIFT

This exercise works the muscles in your thighs, buttocks, and shoulders, while also increasing your core stability. It helps with your flexibility and balance too, as the exercise requires you to center your body weight on one leg for most of the exercise, while moving your other leg through a full range of movement. To make the exercise more difficult, try starting the movement from the raised knee position (**»Step 6**) without pausing in the middle.

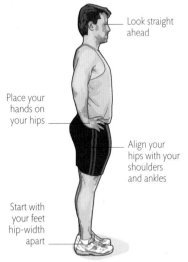

Look straight ahead

Place your hands on your hips

Align your hips with your shoulders and ankles

Start with your feet hip-width apart

1 Stand with your feet hip-width apart, your legs and back straight, and your hands on your hips.

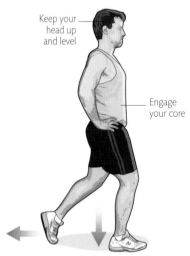

Keep your head up and level

Engage your core

2 Breathe in and lunge backward with your left leg, taking your weight on your right leg as you do so, and bending your right knee slightly.

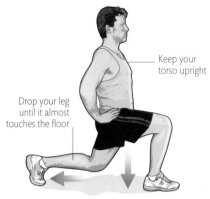

Keep your torso upright

Drop your leg until it almost touches the floor

3 Continue the movement until you are in a full lunge position with your left knee almost touching the floor, or as far as you can comfortably go.

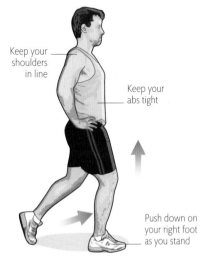

Keep your shoulders in line

Keep your abs tight

Push down on your right foot as you stand

4 Start raising yourself up by straightening your right leg and pushing down on your right foot. Bring your left leg forward at the same time.

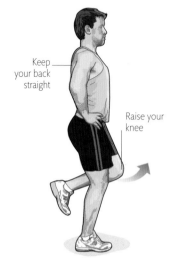

Keep your back straight

Raise your knee

5 Straighten your right leg fully and continue the forward movement with your left leg, pushing through your left knee.

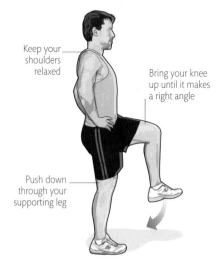

Keep your shoulders relaxed

Bring your knee up until it makes a right angle

Push down through your supporting leg

6 Push forward and up with your left knee until it is at hip height and bent at a right angle. Pause and return to the start position. Repeat for the required number of reps, then switch legs.

100 HIP FLEXOR STRETCH

Your psoas muscles work as hip flexors and can shorten with prolonged sitting, creating a muscle imbalance. Stretching them reduces strain on your lower back.

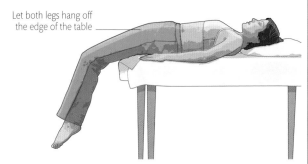

Let both legs hang off the edge of the table

1 Start by sitting on the edge of a firm padded table, with your legs hanging over the side. Then lie back and rest your head on a pillow or folded towel.

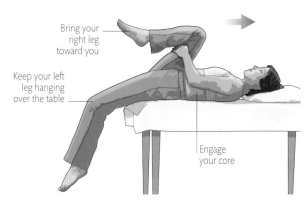

Bring your right leg toward you

Keep your left leg hanging over the table

Engage your core

2 Raise your right leg and bend it at the knee. Grip your thigh and bring your knee close to your chest.

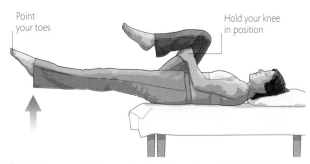

Point your toes

Hold your knee in position

3 Raise your left leg to the horizontal and hold briefly, then relax it, allowing it to drop to achieve a full stretch. Hold for 15 seconds, then return to the start position and switch legs.

101 PSOAS LUNGE

This exercise is an adaptation of a standard lunge that focuses the stretch on your psoas muscle. The key to performing it is to keep your pelvis tucked underneath your torso.

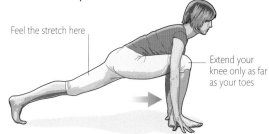

Feel the stretch here

Extend your knee only as far as your toes

1 Lunge your right leg forward, and place your hands on either side of your right foot. Straighten your back leg, and press your left hip toward the floor.

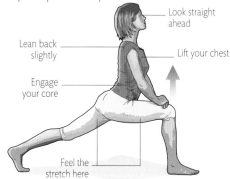

Look straight ahead

Lean back slightly

Lift your chest

Engage your core

Feel the stretch here

2 Tuck your hips underneath you and place both hands on your right thigh. Exhale, lift your chest, and look straight ahead of you.

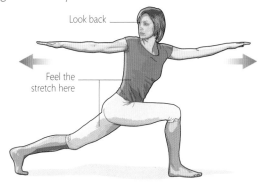

Look back

Feel the stretch here

3 Slowly reach your right arm behind you and twist your torso around, while reaching your left arm out in front of you, so that both arms are extended. Look back in the direction of the twist and hold briefly, then return to the start position. Repeat as required, and switch legs.

102 KNEELING HIP FLEXOR

This exercise will stretch your hip flexor muscles, which may be particularly tight if you spend a lot of time sitting down. Tight hip flexors can cause imbalances around your pelvis and lower back, leading to back pain. If you find your knees hurt during the movement, you can rest them on a cushion or soft pad.

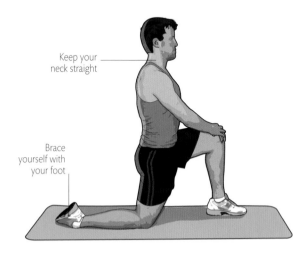

Keep your neck straight

Brace yourself with your foot

1 Kneel on your right knee, with your hands resting on your left knee for balance, so that your right knee is below your shoulders and your head is in line with your back. Keep your back straight.

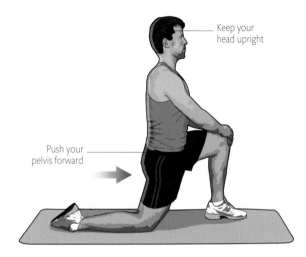

Keep your head upright

Push your pelvis forward

2 Bring your left knee forward and feel the stretch in the thigh of your right leg, but don't extend your left knee over the front of your left foot. Hold the stretch for 15 seconds, relax, and switch sides.

103 PRONE ARM AND LEG LIFT

This exercise strengthens the muscles around your shoulders and along your spine, along with your buttocks and hamstrings. It is especially useful for people who can't kneel properly or have wrist problems and can't perform the kneeling superman exercise (»p.99).

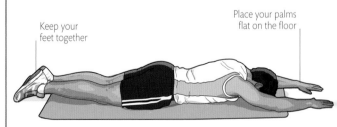

Keep your feet together

Place your palms flat on the floor

1 Lie face down with your forehead resting on the mat. Align your neck and head. Extend your arms in front of you with your palms facing down. Lengthen your torso by stretching your neck away from your body, and contract your abdominals.

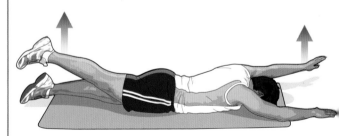

2 Keeping your head in line with your upper back, raise your left arm and your right leg 3–6 in (8–15 cm) off the floor. Hold the movement briefly.

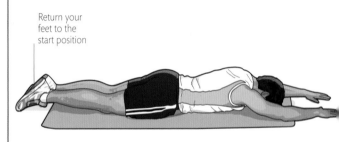

Return your feet to the start position

3 Lower your limbs slowly and with control, and return to the start position. Switch sides and continue to alternate sides until you have completed the required number of reps.

104 **OBLIQUE** CRUNCH

This exercise requires flexibility, stamina, and mobility. It can potentially aggravate some types of back pain, so seek guidance to ensure that it is right for you and that you are performing it with good technique.

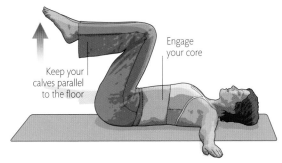

1 Lie on your back with your pelvis in a neutral position, your knees and hips bent at 90 degrees, and your arms outstretched at right angles to your body.

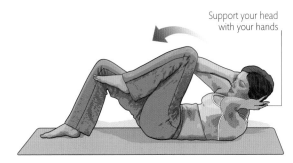

2 With your hands held lightly to the sides of your head, simultaneously bring your left knee and right elbow together, planting your right foot firmly on the floor.

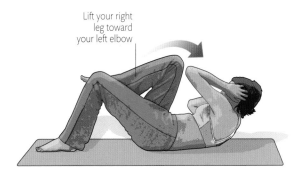

3 Alternate the movement at a steady pace, ensuring that you curl up and rotate your trunk, and avoid pulling your head or neck. Complete the required number of reps before returning to the start position.

105 **SIDE** CRUNCH

Side crunches target the oblique muscles responsible for core strength and trunk stability. They can potentially aggravate some types of back pain, so consult your physical therapist for guidance first.

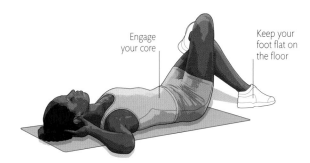

1 Lie on your back with your pelvis in a neutral position, your left leg bent to 90 degrees, and your left foot firmly on the floor. Rest your right leg across your left knee, and place both hands at the base of your head.

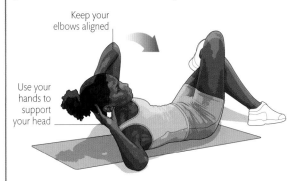

2 Keeping your lower back pressed into the mat, lift your shoulder blades off the floor. Leading with your left elbow, curl your upper body toward your right knee.

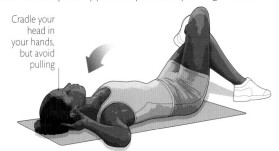

3 Pause briefly, then return to the start position slowly and with control. Repeat until you have completed the required number of reps, then switch sides.

106 CHILD'S POSE

This yoga position gently stretches your spine, hips, thighs, and ankles. If you find the exercise uncomfortable, you can place a rolled-up towel between the back of your thighs and calves.

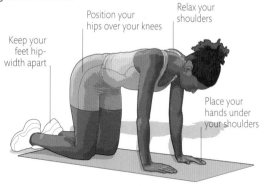

Keep your feet hip-width apart

Position your hips over your knees

Relax your shoulders

Place your hands under your shoulders

1 Kneel on all fours with your hands in line with your shoulders, your fingers pointing forward, and your knees directly below your hips. Keep your back straight and your head in line with it.

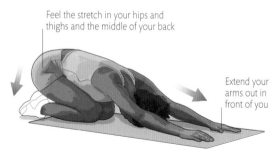

Feel the stretch in your hips and thighs and the middle of your back

Extend your arms out in front of you

2 Keeping your hands in position, slowly lower yourself down onto your heels until your forehead touches the mat. Breathe in and out, and feel the stretch in your body.

VARIATION

This exercise can also be performed with a slight variation to stretch the side muscles of your back. Instead of stretching your arms out directly in front of you, stretch them out diagonally, keeping them parallel as you do so. Hold the position for a few seconds, then repeat on the other side to fully benefit from the stretch.

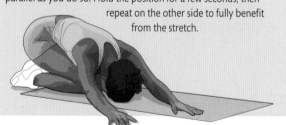

107 SWISS BALL ROLL-OUT

This advanced exercise builds stability and strength in your core muscles because it makes your abdominals and lower back work together. It also strengthens your shoulders.

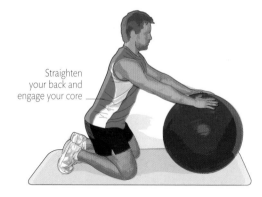

Straighten your back and engage your core

1 Kneel down, resting your hands and lower arms on the top of the ball. Ensure that your back is flat.

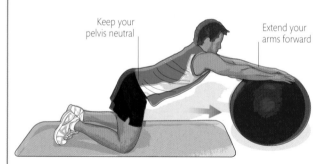

Keep your pelvis neutral

Extend your arms forward

2 Roll the ball forward by extending your arms, and follow it with your upper body as far as you can without arching your back. Use your abdominals to pull the ball back to the start position.

VARIATION

Using a barbell instead of a stability ball is a high-level variation of this exercise, but should only be attempted once you have very good abdominal and spinal control. Kneel with your hands on the bar, shoulder-width apart. Keep your back flat as you roll the bar forward and use your abdominals to pull it back to the starting position.

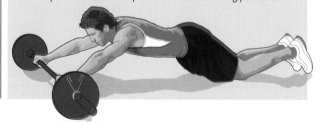

108 SIT-TO-STAND CHAIR SQUAT

Practicing squats helps you develop the habit of using your hips and leg muscles instead of your back. This version is a good confidence-builder, as the chair or box provides a base and you do not have to squat too low.

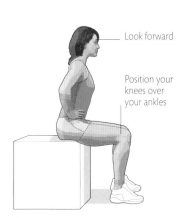
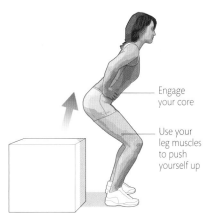
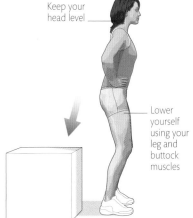

Look forward

Position your knees over your ankles

Engage your core

Use your leg muscles to push yourself up

Keep your head level

Lower yourself using your leg and buttock muscles

1 Sit on the edge of a sturdy box or chair with your knees bent at a right angle over your ankles and your feet hip-width apart. Place your hands on your waist. Inhale.

2 Lean forward from the hips, keeping your back straight. Exhaling, press down through your feet to stand up, and squeeze your buttocks together as you begin to stand.

3 Straighten your knees—without locking them—until you are in a standing position. Pause briefly, then return to the start position slowly and with control.

109 STAND-TO-SIT CHAIR SQUAT

This exercise is almost the reverse of the sit-to-stand version of the chair squat (»above). The arm movement differs slightly, in that your arms are outstretched in front of you, giving you a little more balance.

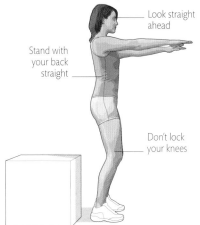
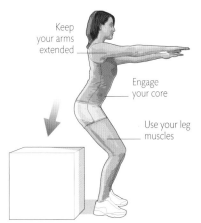
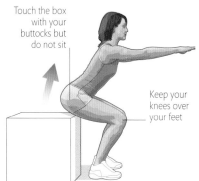

Look straight ahead

Stand with your back straight

Don't lock your knees

Keep your arms extended

Engage your core

Use your leg muscles

Touch the box with your buttocks but do not sit

Keep your knees over your feet

1 Stand in front of a sturdy box or chair with your feet hip-width apart, gently pressing your body weight down through your heels. Raise your arms in front of you and look straight ahead.

2 Pressing down through your heels, inhale and bend at the knees, reaching back with your buttocks and lowering yourself toward the box. Keep your shoulders over your ankles.

3 Continue to bend at the knees until your buttocks touch the edge of the box, but do not sit down. Exhale as you squeeze your buttocks and return to the start position.

GLOSSARY

Abductor A muscle that functions to pull a limb away from your body. See Adductor.

Active range of motion During rehabilitation, the movements you are able to make yourself using muscle strength, as opposed to your *passive range of motion*.

Acute (pain) Pain that comes on suddenly but lasts only a short while and can be treated successfully. See Chronic.

Adductor A muscle that functions to pull a limb toward your body. See Abductor.

Aerobic A process that requires oxygen. Aerobic *metabolism* occurs during long-duration, low-intensity exercises, such as long-distance running and swimming. It is the opposite of *anaerobic*.

Analgesic A drug used to reduce pain.

Anaerobic A process that does not require oxygen. Anaerobic *metabolism* occurs during short-duration, high-intensity exercises, such as in some forms of intensive strength training. It is the opposite of *aerobic*.

Ankylosing spondylitis (AS) A form of spinal arthritis that leads to inflammation and calcification of the ligaments in the *sacroiliac* and invertebral joints.

Antagonistic muscles Muscles that are arranged in pairs to carry out flexion and extension of a joint. See flexor and extensor.

Anterior The front part or surface, as opposed to *posterior*.

Barbell A *free weight* made up of a bar with weights at both ends, long enough to hold with at least a shoulder-width grip.

Bone density The amount of bone mineral in a given volume of bone.

Brachialgia Nerve pain in the arm.

Cervical Relating to the neck area.

Chronic (pain) Pain that persists for a long time and is often resistant to treatment. See Acute.

Coccydynia Pain around the *coccyx*.

Coccyx Bone at the base of the spine.

Cognitive Behavioral Therapy (CBT) A psychological approach that is used to explore and modify how your thoughts influence your perception of pain and your situation.

Cool-down A period after completion of a training session designed to help return your body to its pre-exercise state.

Core The central part of your body, mainly the stomach and lower-back muscles, but also including the pelvis, chest, and upper back.

Core stabilizers Deep trunk, abdomen, paraspinal, and *pelvic floor* muscles. These muscles provide support to your lower back.

Corticosteroids Hormones administered by injection, cream, or tablets, for example to reduce *inflammation*.

CT (Computerized Tomography) scan A type of scan that builds a three-dimensional picture of the body.

Diaphragm The muscle that separates your chest cavity from your abdomen.

Discogenic pain Pain caused by deterioration of *disks*.

Discography A procedure that uses dye and X-rays to look at your spine and confirm if the disk(s) is/are the source of pain.

Disk A cushionlike pad that sits between each vertebra and acts as a shock absorber. Disks allow your spine to bend.

Disk prolapse/protrusion See herniated disk.

Dumbbell A type of *free weight* made up of a short bar with a weight at each end. It can be lifted with one hand.

Dynamic exercise Any activity in which your joints and muscles are moving.

Erector A muscle that raises a body part.

Ergonomics The design of devices that work with the body to help prevent repetitive strain injuries.

Extensor A muscle that works to increase the angle at a joint, such as straightening your elbow. It usually works in tandem with a *flexor*.

Facet joint A small joint that connects each vertebra with the vertebra directly above and below it, providing stability to the spine.

Facet joint strain Pain that occurs when a facet joint is suddenly twisted or jerked.

Flexor A muscle that works to decrease the angle at a joint, such as bending your elbow. It usually works in tandem with an *extensor*.

Form The correct posture or stance used when performing exercises.

Fracture A break in a bone, ranging from minor cracks to serious breaks.

Free weight A weight—usually a *barbell* or *dumbbell*—not tethered to a cable or machine.

Gluteus medius dysfunction Strain in the buttock muscles that hold the pelvis stable.

Head (of a muscle) The point of origin of a muscle.

Herniated disk When a portion of a spinal disk ruptures and bulges outside its normal position, and may press on the nerve roots of the spine.

Hypermobile joint A joint that is loosely held together because the *ligaments* are either naturally lax or have been overstrained (which can lead to *instability*).

Hypomobile joint A joint that moves less than it should, sometimes caused by shortening of the muscles attached to the joint.

Inflammation Swelling, pain, and redness of an area of the body as a response to a harmful stimulus.

Instability Slackening of the ligaments caused by narrowing and tears in a disk.

Isometric A form of training in which you contract your muscles without moving your body or any limbs.

Isotonic A form of training in which your muscles work against a constant resistance.

ITB (Iliotibial Band) A tough group of fibers running along the outside of your thigh that primarily works as a stabilizer of the hip in standing, walking, and running.

Lactic acid A waste product of *anaerobic* respiration. It accumulates in your muscles during intense exercise and is involved in the chemical processes that cause muscular cramp.

Lateral Positioned toward the outside of your body. Movement in the lateral plane refers to a side-to-side movement.

Ligament A tough and fibrous connective tissue that connects your bones together at the joints.

Lumbar Relating to the lower-back area.

Metabolism The sum of all your body's chemical processes (anabolism and catabolism).

Mineral Inorganic elements that are essential for normal body function and must be included in your diet.

Mobility exercise An exercise that helps you maximize the movement of your joints.

MRI (Magnetic Resonance Imaging) A type of scan that reads the molecular structure of your body to form an image to aid diagnosis.

Muscular tension Tensing your muscles, a normal response to stress; a major cause of back pain.

Musculoskeletal Affecting both the muscles and bones.

Neuropathic Relating to pain caused by abnormal processing of nerve signals due to damage or dysfunction.

Neutral spine position The most efficient posture in standing or sitting, or the mid-range position of a joint or region of the spine.

Osteoarthritis A degenerative disease in which the body suffers a loss of cartilage, leading to stiff joints.

Osteoporosis Weakening of the bones caused by loss of minerals, especially common in women after menopause.

Pain-relief medication Different medications have different functions, such as reducing pain by reducing inflammation, but all produce the result of limiting your experience of pain in the body.

Passive range of motion The movements a physical therapist or helper is able to make with parts of your body while supporting their weight. See Range of motion.

Pelvic floor The area of muscle located in the lower part of the abdomen and attached to the pelvis.

Piriformis syndrome Irritation of the sciatic nerve by tightening of the piriformis muscles that rotate the hip.

Plyometrics Exercises that aim to improve the speed and power of movements by training muscles to contract more quickly and powerfully.

Posterior The back part or surface, as opposed to *anterior*.

Proprioception The term used to describe the information originating from joints, tendons, ligaments, and muscles that is sent to the brain to provide information about joint position, direction, and pressure.

Range of motion (ROM) A term used in disk therapy, this is the movement a joint is capable of in every direction.

Regimen A regulated course of exercise and diet designed to produce a predetermined result.

Rehabilitation The process of recovering fully from an injury, often with the assistance of professionals.

Repetition (rep) One complete movement of a particular exercise, from start to finish and back.

Resistance training Any type of training in which your muscles work against resistance, provided by a weight, an elastic or rubber band, or your own body weight.

Rest interval The pause between sets of an exercise that allows muscle recovery.

Rupture A major tear in a muscle, tendon, or ligament.

Sacroiliac joints The two joints located at the base of the back on either side of your spine between the sacrum and the ilia (hip bones).

Sacroiliac strain Damage to the ligaments supporting the *sacroiliac joint*, usually caused by a heavy fall or a blow to the bottom of the back.

Sciatica Nerve pain in the leg.

Scoliosis Curvature of the spine that causes it to twist to one side.

Sensorimotor Relating to processes involving the communication between brain and muscles via the nerves.

Set A specific number of *repetitions*.

Skeletal muscle Also called striated muscle, this type of muscle is attached to your skeleton and is under voluntary control. Contracting your skeletal muscles allows you to move your body under control.

Smooth muscle A type of muscle found in the walls of all the hollow organs of your body which is not under voluntary control.

Spinal stenosis Narrowing of the spinal canal due to bony spurs developing on the vertebrae which protrude into the spinal canal.

Spondylolysis Occurs when a defect in a vertebra develops into a fracture. The vertebra is then at risk of slipping out of line with the vertebrae adjacent to it, leading to spondylolisthesis.

Sprain An injury sustained by a *ligament* that is overstretched or torn.

Stabilizers Small muscles close to the spine that hold the vertebrae or spinal region in alignment for static posture or while dynamic movements are being performed.

Static exercise An exercise in which you hold one position.

Strain An injury to muscle fibers caused by overstretching.

Swiss ball A large, inflatable rubber ball used to promote stability during exercise. Also known as an exercise ball.

Tear A rip in, for example, a muscle.

Tendinopathy Painful *tendons*, often resulting from overuse while doing repetitive actions.

Tendon A type of connective tissue that joins your muscles to your bones.

Thoracic Relating to the chest and back between the neck and *lumbar* regions.

Torticollis An acute stiff and painful neck which makes turning your head sideways difficult and painful. It is often triggered by lying or falling asleep in an awkward position. Also known as "wry neck."

Traction A technique used to straighten or realign bone fractures into a permanent position, or to relieve pressure on the spine and skeletal system.

Warm-up A series of low-intensity exercises that prepares your body for a workout by moderately stimulating your heart, lungs, and muscles.

Whiplash An injury in the neck area following an acceleration-deceleration force, usually as the result of an indirect impact.

Wobble board Circular in shape with a flat top and hemispherical underside, this piece of equipment is used to promote good balance, and to improve your *core* stability.

INDEX

ACKNOWLEDGMENTS

AUTHORS' AND PUBLISHER'S ACKNOWLEDGMENTS

The authors would like to acknowledge the valuable contributions of learned colleagues of The British Institute of Musculoskeletal Medicine and the International Spine Intervention Society for their collective years of experience and study in diagnosis and management of spinal pain. The authors would also like to extend their grateful thanks to their patients.

The authors and publishers would like to thank the following people and organizations for their generous help in producing this book.

For modeling:
Emily Hayden; Eva Hajidemetri; John Tanner; Annie Hajidemetri; Gareth Jones; Scott Tindall; Mary Paternoster; Sam Bias Ferrar; Anne Browne; Chris Chea; Louise Cole; Sarah Cookson; David Doma; Amanda Grant; Michelle Grey; Anouska Hipperson; Elizabeth Howells; Christopher James; Gunilla Johansson; Megan Lolls; Zoe Moore; Sean Newton; Caroline Pearce; Yasmin Phillips; Jamie Raggs; Lucy Shakespeare; Rufus Shosman; William Smith; Kirsty Spence; Sheri Staplehurst; and Sally Way.

For use of facilities:
Dr. Eric Ansell at 999 Medical and Diagnostic Centre.

For equipment:
Paul Margolis of Margolis Office Interiors Ltd (www.margolisfurniture.co.uk) for supplying the ergonomic chair.

For reference photography:
Nigel Wright, XAB Design; Gillian Andrews; Keith Davis; Phil Gamble; Eva Hajidemetri; Cobalt ID; Russell Sadur; and Graham Atkins-Hughes.

For illustrations:
Philip Wilson; Debbie Maizels; Phil Gamble; Mark Walker; Debajyoti Dutta; Mike Garland; Darren R. Awuah; and Jon Rogers.

For additional material and assistance:
Dr. Sue Davidson; Margaret McCormack (indexer); Scott Tindall; Derek Groves; Glen Thurgood; Len Williams; the British Weightlifting Association (BWLA); Scarlett O'Hara, Nicky Munro, Hugo Wilkinson, Georgina Palffy, Kingshuk Ghosal, Suneha Dutta, and Rebecca Warren (editorial); Joanne Clark, Katie Cavanagh, Govind Mittal, and Deep Shikha Walia (design); Ben Marcus and Balwant Singh (pre-production); Mandy Inness (production); and Shanker Prasad (CTS).

SAFETY INFORMATION

Users of this book should not consider the information, advice, and guidelines it contains as a substitute for the advice of medical professionals, accredited physical therapists, and other registered practitioners.

Do not attempt self-diagnosis or self-treatment for serious or long-term problems without consulting a medical professional or qualified practitioner. Do not undertake any self-treatment while you are undergoing a prescribed course of medical treatment without first seeking professional advice. Always seek medical advice if symptoms persist, and do not exceed any recommended dosages of medication without professional guidance.

All physical activity involves some risk of injury. Participants must therefore take all reasonable care during their rehabilitation and maintenance training. Any treatment or rehabilitation program should always be carried out under the guidance of the appropriate professionals.

The publishers of this book and its contributors are confident that the exercises described herein, when performed correctly, with gradual increases in resistance and proper supervision, are safe. However, readers of this book must ensure that the equipment and facilities they use are fit for the purpose, and they should adhere to safety guidelines at all times. They should also ensure that supervisors have adequate insurance and relevant, up-to-date accreditations and qualifications, including emergency first aid.

The publishers, the members and representatives of the British Medical Association (BMA), the consultant editors, and the contributing authors of this book take no responsibility for injury to persons or property consequent on embarking upon the advice and guidelines included herein.